52 WAYS
TO
TRANSFORM
YOUR HEALTH
One Step at a Time

PATTI BOWMAN, CN

Silver Linden Press

Salem, Oregon

52 Ways to Transform Your Health One Step at a Time

Disclaimer

The ideas and suggestions in this book are not intended as a substitute for consulting with your physician. All matters regarding your health require medical supervision. The information and opinions in this book are for educational purposes only, and are not intended to treat, cure, diagnose, or prevent disease

ISBN: 978-0-9981354-4-1
Library of Congress Control Number: 2017912448

Editing by Cherie Buletza
Book Cover Design by Susan D. Johnson
Front cover image by © Olga Demchishina
Formatting by Amit Dey

Printed and bound in USA
First printing

Published by Silver Linden Press
Salem, Oregon USA
healing_pathways@msn.com

Visit Website at www.authorpattibowman.com

Dedication

To Dr. Deb Riekeman, whose skill and deep caring inspired me. You are a true healer and blessing to my life. Thank you.

And to my family and friends, who have had to listen to more about nutrition and health from my mouth than they *ever* wanted to know, and yet were always a source of encouragement. Thank you, dear ones, for your patience and tolerance.

Invitation from the Author

Are You Ready to Make Healthier Choices?

This step by step book will help you take charge of your own health. Here are some **FREE** resources to help you on your journey:

Get a list of things you can eat before bed that will help you sleep and not gain weight. Find it here: https://www. authorpattibowman.com/free-download/

Download a gluten free muffin recipe created by the author. This recipe contains no gluten, dairy, soy, or corn. https:// www.authorpattibowman.com/free-muffin-recipe/

Grab this checklist of the "52 Steps" in this book, to help you plan your transformation to a healthier you! https:// www.authorpattibowman.com/free-checklist-pattis-book/

Enjoy!

Acknowledgments

I am so grateful to the experts who gave of their time and knowledge to enrich this book through interviews and videos: Brad Yates, Cheri Owen, Dr. Bruce Fife, Dr. Brent Smith, and Dr. Manuela Terlinden. I appreciate you very much! A special thank you to the parents of Lincoln, for allowing his wonderful contribution.

I wish to acknowledge my editor, Cherie Buletza, and my cover designer, Susan D. Johnson, for their skill and support of my projects. I could not do this without you!

Special thanks to Tamara Monosoff, my guide throughout this process of bringing a print book to life. Your creativity around "birthing" a book amazes me! You believed it was possible when I doubted.

I have the most amazing family and friends who cheer me on! Thank you for being in my corner.

Message to Readers

This book is interactive! I am delighted to show you how to bring it to life. All the QR (Quick Response) codes throughout the book can be scanned with your Smartphone or iPad to watch the videos that were created especially for you.

The health practitioners featured here have shared from their expertise to help you go a little deeper on several of these "52 steps". Each of the videos is about two minutes long. After you hear their messages, I hope you are even *more* inspired and motivated to step in the direction of optimal health for yourself and your family.

How to Scan the QR Codes in This Book

Step 1: Download a **FREE** QR code reader onto your Smartphone or iPad by searching the App Store.

Step 2: Tap the app once it has downloaded to your phone. This will open up the Reader. Hover over the code you wish to scan, and the camera will automatically take a picture of the QR code. Then your phone (or iPad) will be directed to the respective web page on authorpattibowman.com that contains each video message.

Enjoy!

Table of Contents

Introduction

New Beginnings

Congratulations! By purchasing this book, you have taken the first step toward your best health ever.

I often ask my clients if they are "baby-step" people or "jump-in-the-deep-end-of-the-pool" people. By asking this, I am trying to figure out how fast they want to move in making healthy lifestyle changes. So far, I have had only "baby-step" people. So I wanted to design the information in this book for you. We all have to go at our own speed. All those baby steps add up to a lot of territory covered, as long as you keep stepping. If you are eager, one step each week will bring the transformation you are looking for in one year. Some steps will feel bigger than others.

I recommend that you read this book all the way through first. There is a checklist at the end of the book. Check off the steps you have already taken. Then make a list of all your bodily complaints. Yes, every ache, pain, and pimple! Add to the list as you think of more things. Don't forget the mental things that are going on, too. A good memory is just as important as a good night's sleep. So is a happy mood. This baseline is important. Once people start feeling great, they often forget how bad it was when they started.

Now decide where you want to start, how often you want to try a new step, and when you want to finish. Yes, you need a plan. Some of these ideas will open up your mind. Some will open your heart. Some will put you in touch with your feelings. Some will strengthen your body. I hope you will give them all a try. Experiment! You can always go back to the old way of doing things.

I recommend you do this with a spouse, friend, or group of friends. It really helps to have others cheer you on, and hold you accountable. Besides, it is more fun that way! We all need encouragement, especially when we are starting a new adventure. Let's get started!

Watch Video: Patti Bowman, CN, introduces the book

....

https://www.authorpattibowman.com/52-ways-intro/

Step One

Step One

First Things First-Smoking

Tobacco is first on my list. If you don't smoke, you can skip this step. Smoking (or chewing) is not good for your health. Most people know that it will kill you, eventually, but some people still smoke. I do not understand this powerful addiction, but there are lots of people who do.

I interviewed my friend, Cheryl Owen, R.N. As a Registered Nurse, she has had years of experience as an Educator, Trainer, Facilitator, and Smoking Cessation Counselor. Her first suggestion was the American Lung Association website. You can type in your zip code or State and find classes in your area. According to americanlungassociation.org, "Freedom from Smoking"® is still the leading smoking cessation program for adults. This program gives you the resources to quit within a supportive environment. That sounds like a good place to start!

Your medical doctor may know about other resources in your community, such as public health classes or hypnotherapists who specialize in smoking cessation. Cheryl suggests you try again to quit, even if you have tried before. She states, "This isn't easy and you may need to try several times before you succeed."

People using tobacco, do have nutrient deficiencies. So while you are going through a tobacco cessation program, eat more fresh fruits and vegetables. It will help. Smokers usually can't taste or smell their food. That makes eating not nearly as much fun. It's a process. Food **will** begin to taste better. Exercise also helps by increasing oxygen in your body. Go for it! By quitting, you give yourself a wonderful gift. And you make the world a better place.

Step Two

Just Say "No" to Soda

This next step will feel more like a leap to some of you. I am focusing on soda pop. Soda, pop, colas, soft drinks, (depending on what part of the country you live in) have become part of American culture. It is sprouting in other cultures, too. Soda is almost an icon of the Western world, and it's killing us. We die slowly, so not too many people are noticing. This is a good thing for the soda industry. It reminds me of cigarettes. Those kill you slowly, too. Only with soda pop, you don't smell so bad and can still take a deep breath. How much it discolors your teeth, I don't know. With tobacco, some people quit after the surgeon general put a warning label on the cigarette packs, saying they were bad for your health. In time, there will be a warning label on a can of soda, but why wait for that? Right now, you can just say "no." Drink water instead.

Soft drinks are very hard on the body. The acid in them makes it difficult for your body to regulate pH. Your blood prefers to be slightly alkaline. So your body will buffer the acid, usually with minerals. Most people are low in minerals anyway, due to the fact that our soils are lacking minerals, so the body withdraws minerals from your bones. This is not a good thing for growing children or adults. No one wants osteoporosis later in life. So just say "no."

Drinking soda helps you gain weight. Oh, you drink diet pop, you say? Even people who drink the diet drinks, gain weight. Yes, studies have been done. The weight comes on slowly, about 10--12 pounds a year. And on top of that, aspartame, the artificial sweetener in most diet sodas, is a neurotoxin. Neurotoxins kill your brain cells. They sort of excite them to death. I don't know about you, but I like my brain cells and would like to hold onto them. I want to avoid dementia in my future. These sodas are addictive. Whether it's the sugar, the caffeine, or the artificial sweeteners, yes, they are addictive. Soda pop has absolutely no nutritional value! Is there anything of value in sodas? Well, I understand that colas are useful in cleaning engines.

If you would never consider smoking a cigarette, think of soda pop in the same way. Never drink one. Think of it as a liquid cigarette and just say, "**No!**" Stopping, due to the addictive nature of sodas, will not be that easy. Some people can go cold turkey. Most will have to taper off. Just do it! Your current and future health depends on it. Do NOT switch to sports drinks. Read the ingredient labels. They are mostly sugar-water. They, like sodas, will dehydrate your body. Drink water---w-a-t-e-r.

"But I don't like water," you say? Of course you don't. Water does not taste like soda. You have to re-train your body to like water. Your body will complain at first. Then it will settle in to great relief.

Count up how many sodas you drink in a day, then delete one each day until you are down to one. With that last one, measure out 8 ounces, then 6 ounces, then 4 ounces, then 2 ounces, and then you are done. Carry water with you everywhere you go. Add lemon juice to it, if it helps. Cutting down slowly is a good plan. Just make sure you have a plan, and a date when you will stop. Remember, this is an addiction. Stopping is not easy. But it is possible. You **can** do it! This will make a **huge** difference in your overall health! Share your plan with a friend who will cheer you on and hold you accountable.

Step Three

Dance!

With the first two steps, I was asking you to delete something from your life: tobacco use and drinking colas/soda pop. In this step, I want you to add something—exercise. Some of you already do that. You are ahead of the game. For those of you who would rather sit on the couch or in front of the computer, a change in lifestyle is needed.

Most people think of exercise as a way to lose weight. But it doesn't always work that way. Exercise often makes you hungry. Don't let that stop you. Start to move anyway. Moving gets oxygen to all your cells. Plenty of oxygen means healthier cells! Exercise, stretching, and weight training give you more flexibility and better balance. Exercise moves your lymph. Your lymphatics are like the sewer system of your body. But there is no "heart" to move everything around and keep it flowing. Muscle action moves the lymph.

So does deep breathing, which you should be doing when you exercise.

At the end of a stressful day, exercise is a great way to relieve that stress. You will get a boost of serotonin, that "feel good" hormone. Regular exercise prevents depression. Most people who exercise regularly also sleep better. Regular exercise also protects your brain from dementia. This is a win-win all the way around!

Walking for 30 minutes, 3--5 times a week is all it takes. And if you can't find 30 minutes, take 10. Some people do more moving if they can break up their 30 minutes into two or three sections. Ten minutes of stretching or yoga can totally clear your head! Each person has to figure out what exercise they enjoy doing and when and how to fit it in. Your **entire** body will benefit! And after you exercise, drink water. No soda pop or sports drinks. You deleted those from your life, remember?

Some people hate exercise. They feel worse afterwards. If you are one of those, please see a nutritionist or naturopathic doctor. Your adrenal glands may be exhausted. You might really benefit from some nutritional support. Being active is supposed to be fun. Activity helps us enjoy our lives. Remember, you don't have to go for a run. You don't even have to join a gym. You can walk. Find a friend who will walk with you. You can start with a slow walk. When you walk outside, you get to enjoy nature at the same time. Noticing the beauty around you can really lift your spirits. Listen to your body. Go at a speed that feels good to you. Enjoy the dance!

Step Four

List What You Love

Everyone is encouraged to do this activity. You are going to make a list of all the things you love to do. Sometimes life is so busy, that we don't find time to do things we love to do. After awhile, we forget what those things are. Your list will be a great reminder. So pull out a sheet of paper, (or use some other form of technology), and spend the next five minutes writing them down. **Go!**

You may be surprised at how many things on your list are free, or close to it. Now, do one thing on your list. No excuses. **No excuses!** You will feel better. Getting healthy is all about feeling better. If we don't take time to do those things we love, life loses its luster. Carve out some time and then keep it up. Sometimes you may find an hour, sometimes only 15 minutes, but do it! If you make time to do something that you love every day, then you have a good reason to become healthier—you get more time to do what you love! This is supposed to be fun, by the way. When we increase our enjoyment in life, everything looks better. You can do it. I dare you!

Watch Video: Patti Bowman, CN, talks about Step 4

https://www.authorpattibowman.com/step-4-love/

Step Five

Sit Down and Chew

Every cell in your body needs to be nourished in order to function at its best. Your cells are nourished by the food you eat. I know this sounds way too simple, but Americans have actually forgotten this connection. We think that if our stomachs register "full," then we are covered. So we keep eating, but our cells are starving. That's because we have to absorb the nutrients for the system to work. Now the body has a lot of checks and balances to make up for our ignorance and "hurry" attitude. But that can only carry us so far. Then the body starts to complain. Digestion is not very exciting (unless you are a nutritionist). But it is so very important!! Without proper digestion, you cannot nourish those billions of cells. So here are some simple tips for those of you who really don't care how the system works.

Sit down. This action alone gives your body a clue that you are not in a hurry. That you are ready to relax. (No more standing up over the sink). Relaxation is most important for good digestion. Eating in your car does not count. Neither does eating in front of the TV or computer. Sorry. In order for your body to digest properly, you have to be in a restful, relaxed state of mind. Eating during a business meeting is just not going to cut it. I know you like to multi-task, but this is not the time. (I can't change company habits, but you can at least recommend a copy of my book!) If you have to eat at your desk because there is no place else to go, then post a picture that you love in your space and focus on that while you eat. Or switch work spaces with a friend so you won't be tempted to work and eat.

Chew. It amazes me how many people "inhale" their food! Chewing is the first step in digestion. It not only starts the digestion of carbohydrates, but it triggers other digestive juices to get ready for the meal. Besides, tasting food is part of the joy of eating! It is not about filling up your "tank." It is about savoring the moment. It's about gratitude for this culinary delight! Okay, that may be stretching it for some of you. If you wonder how well you chew, try this experiment. Don't drink anything during your meal. Drink water at the end. Trust me. You will have to chew. Your stomach will thank you for learning this skill.

Focus on the food. Real food, fresh food, delicious food! What a treat!! Focus on the food and all those delicious feelings while you eat. Focus on the love that went into preparing it. Food made with love is much more nutritious! (Ahhhhh…I can hear your cells saying "thank you!")

For the next month, make it a point to sit down when you eat, chew your food well, and focus on the food. I think you will find it life-changing. (And I mean that in a good way.)

Step Six

Label Hunting

You are in the grocery store. You are surrounded by bright colored bottles, boxes, and bags. Some of them call out to you, "extra calcium," "low fat," "vitamin C enriched," "zero trans fats," "all natural." Sounds good, doesn't it? Most consumers reach for what sounds healthy. Here is a big tip. . .the front of the container is *advertising!* Let me say that again. . .**The front of the container is advertising!** Food manufacturers spend lots and lots of money on the label to make sure you pick their product. In order to know what is *really* in the product, you must learn how to read the ingredient label. Where is that, you ask? It is usually on the back of the package, sometimes on the side. It is very small print, so bring your reading glasses. In some cases a magnifier is in order. Don't be sidetracked by the nutrition facts list. This is in much larger print, easy to find, and not all that helpful. I rarely use it.

If you want to be a savvy consumer, learn how to decipher the ingredients. It takes some skill, but you can do it. One important thing to know is that the ingredients are listed in descending order by quantity. Whatever the product has the most of is listed first. So if this product has more sugar than anything else, "sugar" will be listed first. But don't stop there. Manufacturers do not want you to know how much sugar is in their product. You might not buy it. So they stretch it out throughout the ingredient list. First you may read sugar, then later honey, then corn syrup, then maltodextrin, then rice syrup. "Sugar" may be listed 4 or 5 times.

If you see a lot of ingredients that you don't recognize, or can't pronounce, consider putting the food item back on the shelf. As you continue with the steps in this book, I will teach you more about reading ingredients. In the meantime, go into your kitchen cupboard and practice. Look at the advertising. Then look for the ingredients. Compare. That "all fruit juice" you bought may not have as much fruit in it as you thought.

Watch Video: Patti Bowman, CN, talks about Step 6

https://www.authorpattibowman.com/step-6-labels/

Step Seven

High Fructose Corn Syrup

HFCS is short for "high fructose corn syrup." In a nutshell: HFCS makes you fat. Your body gets tricked into wanting to eat more while you store more fat. It is **not** natural, no matter what the advertisers say. This product is designed by humans. Yes, it does come from corn. Corn used to be natural, until it was genetically modified. And about 90% of the corn on the market **is** genetically modified. HFCS is used in nearly all processed foods. Manufacturers love it. It is cheap, extends shelf life of products, mixes easily, and even helps to prevent freezer burn. It is used in most soft drinks. A lot of breads have it included because it keeps them soft.

Yes, there is fructose in fruit. But when you eat an orange, you also eat minerals and vitamins that all work together to metabolize that orange. High fructose corn syrup can raise your triglycerides, your blood pressure, and your resistance to insulin. Eating oranges won't do that. Become an avid label reader and you will understand what I mean when I say that HFCS is in *everything*. Recently, because consumers are becoming better informed, food manufacturers are changing their labels. You may see the words "fructose" or "fructose syrup." It's just another way of saying HFCS. Be wise and delete this item from your diet.

Step Eight

Appreciation

It is time to make another list. On a sheet of paper, or other appropriate device, write down all the things you appreciate about yourself. Spend at least 5 minutes. This list is something for you to keep, so make sure you save the information. It is easier for most people to appreciate others than themselves. Generations ago, if you appreciated yourself, it was considered bragging. Bragging was seen as not a good thing. Ideas changed. We now realize that people thrive when they are appreciated. Do not wait for someone else to appreciate you. Start now to appreciate yourself. It is good for your health.

Learn to accept a compliment. Listen. Take it in. Say "thank you" even if you don't believe a word of it. Don't discount it. The compliment was offered graciously, so accept it graciously.

When you practice appreciating yourself more, you will find that you appreciate others more. When you give compliments, start your sentence with the word "I" rather than "you." "You look beautiful" is much easier to discount than "I think you look beautiful." When you say, "I think," you are giving your opinion, which carries more weight. It is easier to discount someone's statement, rather than their opinion. If you've never done that before, try it and see what you think. I find it amazing how people respond differently.

When you feel "down," pull out your list and remember all the things you appreciate about yourself. It could make your day.

The more we appreciate ourselves, the more people will appreciate us. Appreciation feels really good. We all want to feel really good!

Step Nine

MSG

MSG is short for monosodium glutamate. It is added to food by the food industry as a flavor enhancer. This means that without the MSG, the food would not taste as good and you would probably not buy it. What you may not know is that MSG is a neurotoxin or excitotoxin. Those are big words for "it kills your brain cells." Yes, really, it excites them to death. MSG can be found in a lot of processed foods, including things people buy for quick meals for kids—like soup. It is also found in baby food. Years ago, someone complained about it being in baby food. The baby food industry said they would take it out. Some did. Some just disguised it. So even though you have polished your label reading skills, you have to look for other "words" where MSG is hidden, in order to totally avoid it. As for me, I like my brain cells and would like to keep them. If you would like to keep yours, watch labels for things like: hydrolyzed protein, calcium caseinate, yeast extract. According to Russell Blaylock, MD, these always contain MSG. Not only that, but malt flavoring, broth, stock, natural flavoring, seasoning, and spices, frequently contain MSG. Carrageenan, soy protein isolate, and enzymes may contain MSG. This is not an exhaustive list! For more information, you can read Dr. Blaylock's book, *Excitotoxins, the Taste That Kills.*

Just because you don't feel your brain cells dying, does not mean they have escaped. This is an additive you want to avoid, even if you are not sensitive to it. Keep it out of your cupboard.

Step Ten

Sweet Death-Aspartame

Aspartame is an artificial sweetener. (It is sold under the brand names, NutraSweet® and Equal®.) Aspartame is a neurotoxin. Just like MSG, it kills your brain cells, exciting them to death. So, once again, if you like your brain cells, this additive is one to avoid. It has been associated with everything from headaches to brain tumors to MS to neuropathy. Not something you want to give your kids or yourself. Just because you do not notice symptoms, does not mean it is safe for you to use. Aspartame is also addictive. This is what I read, and clients confirm how hard it is to kick the habit.

Most soda pop drinkers will switch to diet pop in order to control weight. It doesn't work. Artificial sweeteners actually help your body to gain weight. That sweet taste in your mouth triggers an insulin surge. But no calories are there.

Your body was expecting them. So your brain signals you to eat. And most people do, slowly adding on the pounds.

Another artificial sweetener is sucralose. (Sold under the brand name, Splenda®.) Sucralose is not a neurotoxin. Neither has it been proven to be safe. Sucralose is advertised as being natural. It isn't. It is a chemical additive that in animal studies was shown to shrink the thymus gland and enlarge the kidneys. But it made it to the market before any large-scale, long-term human studies could prove or disprove those results. So if you are using it, you are in the study.

As scientists do more and more research on the microbiome (the bacteria in your gut), they are finding that sucralose disturbs your gut bacteria, killing off beneficial organisms. That beneficial balance of bacteria and other microbes that you need for proper health is lost.

I find it interesting that when a product contains artificial sweeteners, it is advertised as "sugar free" rather than "artificially sweetened." Sounds better, don't you think? The implication is that "sugar" is bad but the alternative is much better. Americans have definitely fallen for that line of thinking. Advertisers are smart. They know exactly what to say to confuse us. But now, you are smarter. You are reading this book.

For your health's sake, delete artificial sweeteners from your life.

Step Eleven

Journaling

Journaling is a way to get the busy-ness of what's in your head, down on paper. It can help you clarify what you want or need. What does this have to do with health? A lot, actually! Journaling can be a way to express your anger and frustration and get it out of your body. Sometimes it is easier to let go of an issue once it is down on paper. Some people journal just to keep a record of their day. I think journaling is more effective if you get down to the feeling level. It can be amazing what insights flow out of the end of your pen, when you really express yourself honestly.

All you need is a spiral notebook. Be sure and date your entries. No one reads your journal pages, unless you want them to. Spelling is not important. Neither is punctuation, sentence structure, or penmanship. It is really about processing and getting in touch with the "inner you." Caution: if you want to read over your pages at a later date, writing legibly is helpful.

If there is a part of your body that you don't like, write a letter to it. If you are in pain, write a letter to your pain. If you have an organ or a system in your body that is not working well for you right now, write a letter to it. Hold nothing back. Tell it exactly what you think and how you feel. When you are finished, start on a fresh page and have your body part, pain, or organ/system write a letter back to you. This may feel a little weird at first, but if you will just start moving your pen, you may be surprised at what insights you uncover. Insights help us make better choices.

Start a journal and write in it every day for two weeks. You may find you like it. (You may hate it.) Give it an honest trial. Clarity about your life is a great benefit to your health.

Step Twelve

Please Pass the Salt

Most people think that a low salt diet is healthier for you. It depends on the type of salt. There is refined salt and **un**refined salt. Refined salt has two minerals—sodium and chloride. **Un**refined salt contains over 80 minerals. Most of these are trace minerals; but magnesium, calcium, and potassium are included. Eating refined salt all the time provides the body with too much sodium. But the trace minerals in **un**refined salt, offer balance to the body. Our bodies need these minerals, especially when the soil is depleted of so many.

Manufacturers first began refining salt to give it a longer shelf life and because they believed consumers would see the "white" salt as more pure, thus increasing sales. They were probably right about that. To make this "white" salt flow, they put in additives like aluminum. This is not good for your brain or your health. So as you switch to **un**refined salt, it may look really weird to you at first. Some of it is pink and some gray. Some comes in bigger chunks that go into a salt grinder. It won't take long before you get used to the "look," and you will be on your way to better health. You will also feel more comfortable when someone says, "Please pass the salt." If you are still skeptical, read Dr. David Brownstein's book, *Salt Your Way to Health*.

Most grocery stores now carry **un**refined salt. Look in the "health food section." Sea salts are an option. I like Redmond's *Real Salt*. Both are good. Pick one and try it for at least a month. You will be glad you switched.

Step Thirteen

All You Need Is Love

Most people are aware that children (and adults) need love to grow and thrive. "Being in love" is a feeling that makes us "float" as we walk. We are so happy all the time that no one can really ruin our day. Everything goes better with love.

Now take a day or two and listen to the thoughts in your head. "I am so fat!" "My hair never does what I want!" "I wish my thighs weren't so large." "I am such a loser/failure/ geek." "I have so much pain in my knees/back/head." "Why can't my body cooperate?" "I think I am doomed for the rest of my life!" "I wish I had the energy for that!" "I hate getting old!" Do you hear any of these thoughts?

Have you ever had critical bosses? Did you like working for them? Did you find it discouraging to never get anything right? Maybe you looked for another job with a better working environment. You have over 50 trillion cells in your body. They all hear your thoughts. They all respond to your criticism. And they can't exactly leave.

Every cell in your body needs to be nourished with quality food. Every cell also needs your kind thoughts. Everyone cooperates better when they are shown love and acceptance. So make it a habit to send bright beams of love and acceptance to every part of your body, even the parts that give you pain or consternation. Remember, your body has probably put up with plenty of criticism and abuse for years. . .and it is still here. You can thank it for that. Practice accepting yourself just the way you are. Practice, practice, practice! Say nice things to yourself. And when you catch yourself being mean, say you're sorry, and find something nice to say. Be the kind of "boss" that everyone wants to work for. You may just find that pain lessens, you feel younger, and you actually float when you walk.

Step Fourteen

Sweet Sleep

Everyone agrees that sleep is important. We all feel better after a good night's sleep, yet so many people don't want to go to bed. (Not just kids, but adults, too.) Many people take prescribed medications just to get any sleep at all. Those "sweet dreams" seem far away.

Deep sleep allows the body to repair itself. Growth hormones are released, and the immune system is activated. So a good night's sleep does more than just make you more alert during the following day. Sleep needs to be a priority. Pick a time and be in bed by that time. 10:00 pm is recommended. (And that depends on what time you have to get up!) People, who stay up past 11:00 pm, often get a "second wind." They suddenly feel very productive and are up for 2--3 more hours. They don't realize that their adrenal glands kicked in and that is where their "second wind" comes from. This is not healthy.

It is important to create a sleep environment. Your bedroom should be a very relaxing, peaceful place to be. That means, no clutter, no TV, no computer, no electronic stuff. Limit yourself to a lamp and an alarm clock. Have a bedtime ritual that prepares you for sleep. (This does not include, falling asleep in front of the TV.) If you are the kind of person who has trouble turning off your brain at night, try writing down what you plan to do the next day. If something is bothering you, write it down in a journal before you go to bed. If you have a problem that needs solving, write down the problem and leave the paper and pen on the table. (Let your subconscious work on it instead of you.) You might be surprised how you wake up with the answer.

To aid relaxation, avoid alcohol, caffeine, and foods that upset your stomach. Some people are bothered by electromagnetic fields. So stay off the computer and cell phone late at night. A warm bath, deep breathing, tensing and relaxing muscles, and counting blessings are other helpful techniques. Try a protein snack before bed. ("Snack"--- as in small amount. Not a meal.) Sometimes it is just a matter of a new mattress or pillow.

If, nothing works, no matter what you do, get out of bed. Do some physical work like cleaning out the cupboards or mopping the floor. Doing something constructive is better than tossing and turning. Just knowing work is in your future if you don't sleep may be all the motivation you need.

I talk to a lot of people who say, "I'm a night person. I've always been that way." And that may be true. It may also just be a habit. Consider a trial run. Get to bed by ten o'clock every night for a week. See what happens. You might just find yourself more productive during the day. If not, that's okay. Pick a time that allows you to wake up for your day, and feel refreshed. Find your body's rhythm and stick to it. Consistency is important!

Good night. . .sweet dreams. . .and may all your dreams come true!

Step Fifteen

Let's Make a Movie-Visualization

Everyone runs movies in their mind. It's called daydreaming. Visualization is daydreaming with a purpose. In this case, the purpose is to improve your health. Can you picture yourself at your ideal weight? Can you picture yourself doing something you would love to do with a healthy body? Can you picture a part of your body healing itself? People have done amazing things simply by creating movies in their mind first. Your subconscious mind loves pictures. It will take those pictures and begin to create that for you. It's more powerful if you can be "in" the movie, rather than just watching it. You can kick it up another notch by adding feelings. How does it feel to walk across a room wearing that outfit you love? How does it feel when you get to play tennis again? How does it feel to go hiking after your hip has healed? Take some time every day to run these movies—even 5 minutes.

When you first wake up or before you go to sleep, your subconscious mind is the most receptive. Use your imagination. Have fun! You now have permission to stare out the window and daydream.

Step Sixteen

Friends and Neighbors-Local Farmers

I love farmer's markets! There is something fresh and color-ful and exciting about them. You never know what you will find. In my town, the farmer's market has everything from food to crafts to flowers. You can buy a bouquet of tulips or a bouquet of radishes.

Besides walking around in the fresh air and sunshine, you get to meet local farmers. You have the opportunity to ask about their farms. Do they grow organically? Do they use pesticides and herbicides? When do they harvest certain crops? Do they welcome visitors to their farms? You learn about the growing season. You learn about places where you can go pick your own berries. You make connections. Mostly, you connect to the source of your food. And you can teach your children all about it. Visiting your local farmer's market is a great family outing. Poke around and you may also learn about local community gardens. You might want to start a garden of your own.

When you buy local, from people you get to know, you learn about the quality of your food. You support the local economy. You support small farmers who love what they do and love the land they work on. Your food is fresher, tastier, and contains more nutrients---not to mention, a lot of love. It's a win-win situation. Let your kids pick out a new vegetable they haven't seen before and give it a try. It's an adventure!

Watch Video: Patti Bowman, CN, talk about Step 16

https://www.authorpattibowman.com/step-16-farmers/

Step Seventeen

GMOs-What Are They Thinking???

Today, more than 85% of U. S. corn contains a special gene added that allows the corn to produce its own pesticide. That way when bugs eat the corn, they are killed right away. Sounds clever, doesn't it? Except that when **we** eat the corn, we also eat the pesticide. Somehow, that doesn't sound healthy to me. Genetic engineering (GE) is a laboratory process whereby a gene from one species is inserted into another species for a specific result. It is also called genetically modified organism (GMO).

This is not the same as grafting, breeding, or hybridizing. You can breed a dog with another dog and get a new variety. But you cannot breed a dog with a tomato. Basically, that is what genetic engineers are doing. They are crossing species barriers. Sometimes they use viruses or bacteria to insert the new DNA into the plant or animal. The technology is not an exact science, so side effects are impossible to control. This "let's try it and hope for the best" mentality has entered our food supply. (Actually, it has been there for more than a decade.)

Who is protecting the American people?

No one. We are guinea pigs for corporate profit.

According to the *Non-GMO Shopping Guide* website (nongmoshoppingguide.com), these are the current GMO foods on the market: sugar beets (95%), soy (94%), cotton (90%), canola (90%), corn (88%, Hawaiian papaya (more than 50%), plus a small amount of zucchini and yellow squash. And then you have to consider all the products derived from these, like: sugar, soy sauce, soy milk, soybean oil, cottonseed oil, canola oil, corn chips, corn oil, cornstarch, cornbread, high fructose corn syrup, to name just a few. On top of that, these same foods are fed to animals that we eat. So they become a part of the beef, dairy products, pork, chicken, and eggs that are in our diet.

The above mentioned website has some suggestions: 1. Buy organic. 2. Look for the "Non-GMO" label. 3. Avoid the most obvious GMO's by reading the ingredient label. (See previous paragraph for the list.) 4. Use their free shopping guide list to help you choose wisely. Be sure and take note of the long list of pharmaceuticals, which contain genetically modified ingredients. Many of them are for children. Some vitamin companies use soy and corn as fillers. **Learn to read labels!!**

The American Academy of Environmental Medicine (AAEM) considers GE foods a serious health risk. Of the four websites I visited to gather information, I liked the

Non-GMO Shopping Guide best. It was clear and easy to read. Other websites have good information and go into more depth on the subject. First we need to be informed. Second, we need to create a tipping point. According to one website, it only takes 5% of the American public to do this. We have much more power than we think!! If 5% of the American food consumers would change their diets to exclude genetically modified foods, the food industry would consider GMOs a liability and stop using them. Our children and grandchildren are counting on us to leave the world a better place.

Go into your pantry and start reading labels. Which GMO products are included in the foods you now buy? Find an alternative (which means you may need to buy organic) and make the switch.

Chuckles and Chortles

I have a brown monkey. It has a laugh track inside. When I flip the switch, it rolls around on the floor laughing hysterically. If I get down on the floor with the monkey, it's even better. The laugh track has a very realistic sound. It is impossible to hear that laughter and not start chuckling to myself. When I show other people my brown monkey, they always respond with *at least* big smiles. Most start laughing.

Laughter lifts our spirits. Laughter is healing. Laughter brings lots of oxygen into our bodies. Laughter is the most fun way to be healthy: a good joke, a great cartoon, a person doing silly things. We like to be around people who make us laugh. Norman Cousins wrote a book, *The Anatomy of an Illness,* where he talks about how he used laughter as part of a protocol, to heal himself from an incurable disease. All kinds of good chemistry happen in our bodies when we laugh.

Just smiling can shift your attitude. Try it. Plaster a big smile on your face and hold it for 15 seconds. The best time to do this is when you don't feel like it. Even a sarcastic smile will work. You feel so silly doing this that your smile becomes genuine, and you feel just a tiny bit better.

Find your own "brown monkey." If you need a laugh track to get you started, get one. Watch a funny movie, read a funny book, call a funny friend. Every day find something to laugh about. Your health depends on it!

Step Nineteen

Success

At the end of the day, we often focus on our failures. We may have had only one failure, but it is sure to get our undivided attention. All of our successes fade into the background. Why is that? Do we want a day when everything is "perfect?" Maybe. I think that to gain more success, we need to focus on success. So get out a piece of paper or other technological device and make a list. (I like lists. Can you tell?) I want you to list every success in your life that you can think of. Start at the beginning and move forward, or go backwards. You decide. Think of the big events, like: passing that driving test, graduation, your first job. Little things will pop into your head. Maybe you got those thank you notes written, or made that appointment with the chiropractor. Write those down, too. We forget that life is full of little successes. But each one brings us closer to our goal, whatever that is.

We usually celebrate the big events, but not the little ones. I think the little ones deserve a mini celebration, even if we just exclaim, "I did it!"

Keep your list in a handy place. On those days when you feel like you can't do anything right, read your list. Remind yourself of all the things you have accomplished in your life. Wow! You have succeeded in the past, you can succeed now! By shifting your thinking, you feel a little bit better about yourself. And feeling better is what health is all about.

Lincoln—Step 19

Watch Video Message from Lincoln

https://www.authorpattibowman.com/lincoln/

Watch this 17 month old child learning to walk. When he reaches his destination, he squeals, "I did it!" Keep that in mind whenever you reach a goal. Celebrate! Celebrate the big wins and the little ones. Why? Because it feels good! Celebrate even if no one is watching.

Step Twenty

The Facts on Fat

Eating fat is an important part of a balanced diet. Fat gives our food flavor and slows digestion, allowing us to feel satisfied for a longer period of time. For the past 40 years, fat has been discussed as if it were a bad thing, especially saturated fat. We have been misled.

Saturated fat makes up about half of each cell membrane. And we have over 50 trillion cells in our body. We need saturated fat. Our brains are made up of nerve cells that contain a lot of fat. Without a sheath of fat surrounding the nerve cell, our nerve impulses could not move as fast. We need healthy fat.

Cows that run around in pastures, eating green grass, (and are not fed antibiotics and growth hormones), are going to give quality butter. That butter will be high in vitamins A and D. Pigs that run around in the sunshine will make quality

fat (lard), high in vitamin D. Organically grown olives produce quality oil. Olives can be pressed without heat and
therefore remain unrefined. Coconut oil is very saturated. It
is the perfect oil for high-heat cooking, like stir-fry. Because
it is saturated, it is stable and can take the heat without oxi-
dizing (going rancid). It can also be used in baking, like you
would use butter.

The vegetable oils you see in the grocery store all look
and taste the same. That's because they are all refined. Chemical solvents have been used to extract the oil. But fresh oils,
taste and smell like the seeds they come from. Nobody eats
cottonseeds or rapeseeds (canola), so why use the oil? Soybean oil and corn oil come from genetically modified crops
(as well as cottonseed and canola). These oils, all polyunsaturated, can easily become rancid during the refining process.
You would never know because the rancid taste is removed
by the manufacturer. These four oils are most prominent in
processed foods. They are also on the "most-likely-to-be
genetically-modified" list.

I always recommend that people spend money on the best
quality fat. Plants and animals (and people), tend to store
toxins in fat cells. So if you are eating the fat of a plant or
animal, guess what? You get the toxins, too. People always
ask me about those butter spreads, the ones with the clever
names. And I always say, *"Read the ingredients!"* Some of
them do not contain any butter. Some of them contain GMOs.

Organically produced fats and oils are safest. This is
really all your kitchen needs: butter and coconut oil for cooking, eating, and baking, and olive oil to make salad dressings.
Then you can add in organic avocados and organic raw nuts.

If you want to use lard, make sure it comes from healthy pigs and contains no additives. Bacon needs to come from healthy pigs and be nitrite-free.

Bruce Fife N.D.—Step 20

Watch Video Message from Bruce Fife, N.D., Author of *Oil Pulling Therapy*

https://www.authorpattibowman.com/step-20-bruce-fife-n-d/

Dr. Bruce Fife, C.N., N.D., is an author, speaker, certified nutritionist, and naturopathic physician. He has written over 20 books including *The Coconut Oil Miracle,* and *Stop Alzheimer's Now!* He is the publisher and editor of the *Healthy Ways Newsletter* and serves as the president of the Coconut Research Center, a non-profit organization whose purpose is to educate the public and medical community about the health and nutritional aspects of coconut and related foods. Dr. Fife is considered one of the world's leading experts on dietary fats and oils. He is a popular speaker and with his wife, Leslie, travels throughout the world lecturing at health fairs, conferences, hospitals, and spas. He has appeared on hundreds of radio and television programs worldwide. He can be reached at: www. piccadillybooks.com and www. coconutresearchcenter.org.

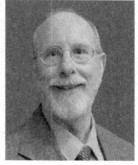

Bruce Fife, N.D.

Step Twenty-one

Trans Fats-No Transfers Please

The subject of fats is very confusing to most people. What does saturated, unsaturated, polyunsaturated mean anyway? And now the new one—trans fats. Well, it's really all about chemistry. Fatty acids (or fat molecules) are made up mostly of carbon atoms and hydrogen atoms. If a molecule (fatty acid) is full of hydrogen, it is saturated (with hydrogen). If any hydrogens are missing—it is **un**saturated. If one pair of hydrogens is missing, it is mono-**un**saturated. If more than one is missing, it is poly-**un**saturated. Didn't help? Moving on.

Every fat contains some saturated fatty acids and some unsaturated fatty acids. Whichever it has the most of, places it in a particular category. For example, coconut oil has 92% saturated fat. So it would fall into the saturated fat category. Lard is 50% monounsaturated fat, 40% saturated fat, and 10

% polyunsaturated fat. So it belongs in the monounsaturated category. Surprised? So was I. Still confused? Moving on.

Saturated fats are great for your health, as long as they come from *quality sources.* Examples are coconut oil, butter, and tallow. Monounsaturated fats are good for your health as long as they come from *quality sources.* Examples are olive oil and lard. Polyunsaturated oils are very fragile. They go rancid easily. (Rancid means spoiled.) They should not be exposed to light, air, or heat. **You should not cook with them!** Flax oil is very, very polyunsaturated. If you choose to use it, buy it in small quantities, keep it refrigerated, and don't heat it.

I am old enough to remember when food processors used coconut oil and palm oil in all ready-made foods. They loved it. It was easy to use and gave the food a longer shelf life. When the "experts" claimed that saturated fats were "bad" and polyunsaturates were "good", food manufacturers had to come up with something else. Hydrogenation was the answer. It allowed them to take liquid oil and make it solid. It's actually quite inventive, except that it totally destroys the oil. Remember chemistry? Polyunsaturated oils are very fragile. They oxidize (which means go rancid) easily. These oils go into high temperature, high pressure reactors when subjected to hydrogen gas. In the process of adding hydrogen to make a more solid fat, some of the hydrogen transfers to the other side of the molecule and you have a trans-fat. This is not a good thing.

Your body does not see these "fake fats" as toxic. It incorporates them into your cell membranes anyway. But the chemistry is wrong. These cells have difficulty communicating. They become dysfunctional.

On the ingredient label, if you read "hydrogenated fats" or "partially hydrogenated fats", you know that *trans fats* are in the product, **no matter what the nutrition facts state!** Food manufacturers know that if their product contains .5 or less of any ingredient **per serving**, they can list it as *zero* on the Nutrition Facts Label. That is why you read ingredients!! There is **no safe limit of trans fats** in the human body.

For those of you "younger" people who have grown up with "no fat, low fat, reduce fat thinking," all this may be hard to swallow. So let's look at the big picture. Forty years ago the American public was asked to change their diet. We were to reduce saturated fat, and start using "healthy" poly-unsaturated fat. And so we did. Has it worked? Do we have less heart disease? Are we healthier? The opposite has happened. We have more heart disease than ever before, and, added to that, more obesity. What is wrong with this picture? I think a second look is in order.

I recommend to everyone to use organic quality fats: real butter (not a butter spread), coconut oil, and olive oil. That keeps it simple. If you have margarine in your house, throw it away!!

Step Twenty-two

Gratitude

Gratitude is a great attitude changer. Try it some time when you are standing in line, or stopped at a red light. Make it a game. How many things can you name before it is your turn? Play the "What am I thankful for?" game with your kids in the car. When your day is going badly, pause and take a gratitude inventory. You will be amazed how your day starts to turn around. Even if you have to force yourself to start, soon it becomes easier and you can think of lots of things to be grateful for. It's easy to get bogged down in problems, but gratitude can really lift your spirits. People, who feel better, are more creative problem solvers.

Consider keeping a gratitude journal. Every night, think about your day and write down at least five things for which you are grateful. Continue this journal every night for 30 days. Maybe it will help to find a "gratitude partner." Find someone who will commit to 30 days. Every morning send an email with your gratitude list from the night before. Not only are you remembering what you are grateful for, but you get to enjoy the gratitude expressed by someone else. It's really fun to look forward to those emails! By focusing on gratitude, your outlook becomes more positive. Positive mental health brings better physical health.

Step Twenty-three

Bring in the Sun

I can still remember being told, when I was a kid, to go outside and get some fresh air and sunshine. It was like taking a vitamin. Fresh air seems to clear the head. These days it is more difficult to find fresh air outside, especially if you live in a city. But we all recognize fresh air when we encounter it, and we tend to breathe deeply.

The inside of our homes can be full of chemicals---from cleaners to chemical scents used to cover up the smells we don't want. Then there is out-gassing from furniture, carpets, and paint. Whatever is green outside, filters the air and gives us back a great supply of oxygen. A living green plant in each room of the house will also help keep the inside filtered.

And then there is sunshine! Our body does make a vitamin when our skin is exposed to the sun—vitamin D. We have been taught to be afraid of the sun for the past two decades, maybe three. Some of you were brought up on sunscreen. Now many Americans are deficient in vitamin D. Our health has suffered. Sunburn is not fun either. We have to have a balance.

Sunlight may be more important to us than just a vitamin. In 1973, John N. Ott published a book called, *Health and Light*. Ott was first known for his time-lapse photography. This work led him into photobiology. Through many of his experiments, he discovered that sunlight entering our eyes affected our health. One of those experiments showed that people working under pinkish light tended to be irritable and have more health issues. Most of us work under artificial light. We look at computers, we drive looking through a windshield, we watch TV, and we wear tinted sunglasses or glasses.

You don't have to "look" at the sun, or even sit in the sun, to benefit from this light. You can sit outdoors in the shade, as long as sunlight can enter your eyes without anything blocking the path of the rays. (Like sunglasses, or any glasses.) Ott believes that the body is thrown out of balance when the eyes do not receive the full spectrum of light.

Because of Ott's work, you can now buy an Ott light to bring full spectrum light into your house. Or, you can just go outside for some fresh air and sunshine! Do it every day, even when it's cloudy.

Step Twenty-four

Affirmations

An affirmation is a positive statement about the truth you wish to see in your life. So if you are overweight and say to yourself, "I am my ideal weight," that can feel really weird and awkward. Tell yourself that you are telling the truth in advance.

Affirmations are a great way to re-program the brain after years of negative talk. You can say them out loud. You can write them. You can make a recording and listen to them. You can use affirmations from books, the Internet, or make up your own. You can take a negative thought and turn it around into a positive one. Take "I am so fat" and turn it into an affirmation. "I am now my ideal weight." Or, "I love and accept myself just the way I am." If there is something that you really want in your life, write an affirmation about that. Affirmations can be used for any subject.

Here are some guidelines for writing your own affirmations: (1) Starting with "I am" is very powerful. (2) Keep it positive. (3) Keep it short. (4) Use the present tense, as if it is happening right now.

If you really want to re-program your brain, write your affirmations every day. Repetition works. When you catch yourself in negative self-talk, switch to an affirmation. Have one already picked out and ready to go. Use affirmations to bring your mind back to a positive place.

Create at least one affirmation. Use it during the day when you are waiting on someone or something. It makes the wait go faster. The more you can feel the good vibes of your affirmation, the better. Your subconscious mind is most alert when you first wake up and just before you go to sleep. Those are great times to use your affirmations. Have fun with it!

Step Twenty-five

The Buzz-Caffeine

Caffeine is a drug. It is a legal stimulant, easy to obtain, socially acceptable, inexpensive; and the possibility of addiction is very high. It is found in coffee, tea, colas, chocolate, sports drinks, and medications. Caffeine affects the central nervous system as well as other organs in the body. Then there are the mental components: better alertness and concentration. That's "the buzz." This is followed by tiredness, anxiety, irritability, jitters, lack of concentration, and depression. Time for another cup of caffeine.

Basically, caffeine puts you in "fight or flight" mode. Your mind is more alert, your blood pressure goes up, respiration increases, the liver releases stored energy, and your appetite diminishes. You become a racing machine. Until the caffeine wears off.

Caffeine uses up your stores of thiamine—vitamin B-1. Without enough thiamine, you can feel depressed, irritable, tired, anxious, forgetful, and unable to concentrate. (Hmmm. . . . sounds like my first paragraph.)

Of course, we can also have clarity of mind, alertness, and energy by eating healthy foods, doing something we enjoy each day, exercising regularly, and getting plenty of sleep. We might even enjoy our lives more if we weren't thrown into "fight or flight" sixteen times a day. It's not that caffeine is "bad." But for some people it is. Some should totally abstain.

If you decide to kick the habit, I recommend that you do it slowly. That way you avoid massive headaches, the major drug-withdrawal symptom. You can either cut down on the coffee little by little, or switch to tea which contains less caffeine. Switch from colas to iced tea, if you are a cold caffeine drinker. Then switch to green tea, which has less caffeine than black tea. While you are doing this, don't supplement your diet with chocolate. (And yes, hot cocoa counts.) At the same time you are cutting down on caffeine, try taking a B-complex vitamin. Before you take a pain killer for that drug-withdrawal symptom, read the label. Make sure it does not contain caffeine.

Most people do not regret kicking the habit. They feel so much better! Then, once in awhile, a little coffee, or tea, or chocolate, tastes really good and doesn't rule their lives like caffeine did before. They are in control instead of the drug.

If you are a caffeine drinker who is already dealing with anxiety, depression, irritability, poor sleep, and/or difficulty concentrating, seriously consider getting totally off caffeine!

Consider it even if you "don't drink that much." Some people are very sensitive to caffeine and need to stay away from it completely. The best way to find out is to do a 30-day caffeine-free trial. First, wean yourself off the caffeine and then start counting the 30 days. Remember, caffeine is addictive. You must give your body time to adjust.

Step Twenty-six

Dreams Do Come True

In previous steps, as you were making a list of your successes, or the things you love to do, you may have gotten in touch with your dreams. These are not your sleeping dreams. These are those wistful thoughts that "maybe, someday. . ."

Make another list. Start it with "I always wanted to. . ." Go back to when you were five years old. Make a list of those dreams, those things that you thought would be so cool to do or to learn or to see. Come forward in time and keep adding to your list. Spend at least 5 minutes.

We are taught at a young age to stop dreaming. We are taught to be practical. We are taught that we are too old to start something. We are also taught that we can't have everything we want. It does not matter how impossible it sounds now, write it down anyway! It is true that our dreams do change. But make sure that you are not just pushing your desires out of the way.

What is keeping you from your dream? What steps would you need to take to realize your dream? If you always wanted to go to college, what is the first step you would need to take? Many times when we have classified our dreams as impossible, but we start taking steps toward them, we find that they just might be possible after all.

Part of a healthy life is to have something to look forward to, something to be excited about. Some call it a purpose, or a goal. Don't give up on your dreams! They matter. You are no longer five. Give yourself permission to dream. Give yourself permission to go after your dream.

As you look at your list, choose one. During the next week, take one step toward that dream. That could be as simple as getting on the computer and doing some research about the dream. You may find a class in your community where you could get more information. You may find that the dream doesn't excite you like it once did. Whatever it is, just take that step.

Watch Video: Patti Bowman, CN, talks about Step 26

https://www.authorpattibowman.com/step-26-dreams/

Step Twenty-seven

Organic vs. Conventional

All food used to be organically grown. Now organic produce carries a sticker. If each piece of conventionally grown produce had a sticker that said, "Sprayed with Pesticides," would you buy it? If you walked into a grocery store and saw a banner over the produce section that said, "Producing This Food Damaged the Environment," would you want to feed it to your family? If a conventionally grown tomato carried a label listing all the chemicals used to grow, store, and ship it, would you want to eat it?

Organic food is not about being a food snob. Organic food contains more vitamins and minerals than conventionally grown food--- often, two or three times more. It also tastes better! Conventionally grown foods are often picked green, shipped over long distances, and ripened with gasses so that they look "good" to the consumer. Animals fed organic feed are healthier and have healthier offspring. And we eat those animals.

On conventional farms, the soil is saturated with chemical fertilizers and pesticides. Chemical fertilizers offer very few nutrients. Plants can grow, but their quality suffers. There are no microbes to help plants absorb vitamins and minerals from the soil, and there are no earthworms.

By eating organically, we protect our children—and grandchildren. Because children are small and still developing, they are more vulnerable when exposed to pesticides and other chemicals. (These cannot just be washed off!) We also protect small family farms. Soil is the foundation of organic farming. Soil health and water health mean health for plants, animals, and people. Runoff from pesticides and herbicides **do** enter our water supply. And then there is the savings in energy. More energy is used to produce chemical fertilizers than to grow and harvest all the crops in the U.S.

Yes, organic food costs more. But for your investment, you get a healthier nation with healthier children, healthier soil, healthier plants, and healthier animals. I think that's a great way to become a powerful force in the world. Right now, according to the United Nations' "Life Expectancy Top 40," thirty-seven countries are healthier than the United States.

We have been conditioned by our cultural food habits to want cheap food. But, really good food is not cheap. Long range thinking is needed here. As an experiment, commit to buying and eating organic food for one week. What is good for us is also good for the planet. And a happy planet gives us healthy food.

Step Twenty-eight

Clutter

Is your house a mess? Do you feel like your life is a mess? What about your health? Clutter can be a constant drain on your energy. You may think you don't "see" it anymore, but it has energy of its own and can cause your energy to slow down to a crawl. You may feel a lack of motivation, even feel depressed. By sorting through the clutter around you, you can become clearer about what you want to do with your life.

People hold onto clutter for different reasons. "But what if I need that?" "I promised myself I would fix that." "But these are all useful items!" "I paid a lot of money for that!!" "Maybe I can wear that again." "My grandma died and I inherited all this stuff." "Oh, yeah, I've been meaning to sort through that." The fear of not having enough, or hurting someone's feelings by giving something away, or hurting the memory of a special person who passed away, causes our houses to fill up with more clutter than we can handle. So we rent places to store it.

Keeping someone else's junk does not honor them. So pick something you love and let that represent the memories you have of that special person. Let the rest go. Make someone else's day! By clearing out the clutter, you allow more space for wonderful things to come into your life. Your thinking will be clearer. You will feel lighter. You might even enjoy living in your house again.

This week de-clutter something in your house or office. It could be a room, a closet, or a drawer. Once you start, it gets easier. You may want to commit to spending thirty minutes each day on de-cluttering. That can keep the job from being overwhelming. Keep at it. If you need more motivation, read Karen Kingston's book, *Clear Your Clutter with Feng Shui.* Mental clarity is a great asset. Emotional clarity can change your life.

Step Twenty-nine

A Toast-Wine

Is alcohol good for your heart? Well, yes, no, maybe, probably not. The wine industry is lobbying hard to convince people that it is good for the heart. And people like to hear that
drinking alcohol is good for them. However, the research is
not convincing. So as not to bore you with research details,
it basically comes down to one researcher saying "yes," and
the next researcher saying "no." Since there is such a con-
troversy, I am wondering who is paying for all this research.

It all started with the French. Beginning in the 1990's, it
was noted that in France, the death rate for cardiovascular
disease was about half what it is in the U.S. And that their
diet is made up of lots of butter, cheese, and meat. It was
also noted that the French drink a lot of wine. Hmmmm.
For some reason, researchers took a giant leap and theorized
that wine could be the benefit. Much research was born.

It became known as the "French Paradox." None of these researchers seemed to notice that the French also eat much less refined sugar (5 pounds a year per person) compared to the U.S. consumption (120 pounds a year per person). And the idea that the French have a slower, more relaxed lifestyle than Americans also went right by the researchers as a possibility. And because the cholesterol theory was already in their minds, it never occurred to them that unadulterated fats might actually BE the protective factor. Or if it did occur to them, they liked the wine theory better.

At any rate, it is not the drink so much as it is the person drinking. Age, gender, diet, genetics, exercise, and drinking patterns, all plays a role in whether you benefit or not. If there are compounds in wine that are beneficial to the body, there are also many that are not. All alcoholic drinks deplete nutrients, especially vitamins C, A, and B complex. But minerals, like zinc and magnesium, are also affected.

Most alcoholic drinks are produced with many chemicals, which preserve, add color, or stabilize the ingredients. Sulfites in wine are an example. And when I say many, I'm talking 20 to 60, **none of which are required to be on the label**. Vineyards are often treated with synthetic fertilizers and pesticides. So if you happen to be one of those people who's heart benefits from drinking wine, your liver, on the other hand, is working very hard to detoxify all those chemicals AND deal with the alcohol. If you choose to drink wine, ask around about organic wines. They do exist.

You do not need to drink wine to have a healthy heart. Just eat plenty of fresh fruits and vegetables, exercise, relax, and reduce your refined sugar intake. I'll toast to that!

Step Thirty

Taste Buds

There are a lot of people who did not like coffee when they first tried it. They "acquired" a taste for it because they were motivated. (And the caffeine "kick" didn't hurt either.) They were motivated because it was so socially acceptable, so much a part of American life, even if it contains no nutritional value. Many people will stop eating healthy food after the first bite, if they don't like it. They do not wait to "acquire" a taste for it.

Most American diets contain two flavors: salt and sweet. Fast food, restaurant food, and "snack food" contain salt and sweet. We are inundated with these two flavors. So it really doesn't surprise me when healthy food is considered "bland." If you want to be healthier, and include healthier choices in your diet, it is important that you give your taste buds a chance to "acquire" a taste for healthy food. Taste buds used to heavy salt and heavy sweet need several weeks to adjust. Then the real flavors of fresh fruits and vegetables come through to delight the palate.

In the beginning, just tell your self, "this is good for me." If, after 3 or 4 times of trying something new, it still doesn't excite you, then move on to the next healthy option. Don't give up. Each fresh vegetable has its own unique flavor. You will never taste that if you are always drowning it in salad dressing. Fresh fruits will begin to taste like dessert if you stop topping them with ice cream. Organic foods usually have better flavor. That is why chefs like to use them. Foods eaten in season usually taste better, too. That is a great time to try something new.

Step Thirty-one

Grass-Fed Beef

You have probably seen labels on beef saying "grass-fed" and wondered what the big deal was. If you do any traveling across the United States, you have seen cattle grazing in fields. So what? Don't all cows eat grass? Yes and no. Most cows graze on grass initially. Then most cows raised to provide your steak or hamburger are fed grain, soy, and corn. (And sometimes parts of each other.) These products are not natural to their digestive systems. For that reason, they develop physical ailments such as bloat and acidosis. Because of this unnatural diet, they must also be fed steroids, hormones, and other chemicals, all of which end up in the meat. These cattle are kept in very small spaces, so must be given lots of antibiotics to prevent disease. Where they live and the cattle themselves are subjected to topical insecticides and antimicrobials. These are also in their feed and residues will show up in your burger. All of this is done to fatten them quickly for market.

Totally grass-fed cows, on the other hand, are allowed to graze on their natural diet of grasses, in an outdoor, more peaceful environment. Cows know how to forage for the healthiest grasses. They are not fed hormones, antibiotics, or steroids. They are treated with respect. And that respect comes back to us in the form of healthy meat with a similar profile to wild game. Bison is another option for healthy meat. They are also totally grass-fed.

Grass-fed beef contains 3-5 times more nutrition than feedlot-raised animals. Grass-fed animals contain more zinc, iron, B-12, CLA (conjugated linoleic acid) and Omega-3, to name a few.

Look for grass-fed beef (or bison) at a farmer's market, health food store, or grocery store. Try it! Ask questions about how the animals are raised and what they are fed. Request tips on how to cook the meat. A happy, healthy cow will provide better nutrition for you.

Step Thirty-two

Forgiveness

I believe that forgiveness is absolutely key to healing. And sometimes people have to spend a lot of time looking deeply within to discover what or who they are mad at and resolve it. Anger can be easily repressed inside us. We can hold onto resentments we aren't even aware of.

A lot of people use the phrase "forgive and forget." I don't believe we ever forget. We can't. It's in our memory banks. But through our forgiveness, we take away the emotional charge. When we think about the event, we feel "neutral." Notice, I didn't say "good." We feel "neutral." We let it go. The event no longer has power over us. We refuse to be burdened by it.

One thing that keeps people from forgiving is the belief that once they forgive, they have to be friends. Not true. When you forgive someone, you give up financing that memory. You let it go. You are no longer putting any of your energy into hiding the memory or keeping it alive. It's over. It's in the past.

Often we don't forgive because we won't make the first move. We think *they* should apologize first. So, we can stay in "junior high thinking" or decide to be an adult, step up to the plate, and do it. If you have had a falling out with someone, now is the time to call that person and patch things up. You will find relief and peace within. You will feel happier and healthier. We hold onto our hurt feelings, hoping the other person can feel our pain. They don't.

Forgiveness is not saying, "It's okay," because sometimes it's **not**. You do not have to confront the person for forgiveness to take place. In some cases that would not be safe at all. But you can write them a letter. This is a form of journaling. You do not send them the letter. You write out your feelings and then shred, burn, or bury the letter. That is your "letting go" moment. When you truly let something go, you don't talk about it anymore. It's over. You do not need to tell anyone you have done this to reap the benefits.

Another way to "let go" is to visualize your anger, resentment, or bitterness as a burden. We carry them around with us every day, draining away our energy. Picture what those burdens look like. Pretend you are carrying them in your arms to a tree and place your "burdens" in the branches of the tree. Trees are strong. They don't judge. Imagine the tree remolding that energy into something useful. Thank the tree and walk away. Forgiveness is emotional housecleaning. It lets us make room for the good we desire.

Take some quiet time and sit comfortably in a chair. Ask yourself, "Is there anyone I need to forgive?" Wait quietly. If some incident or person pops into your head, get in touch with your feelings about that. Sit down with your journal and write them a letter. You may choose to call them. Do whatever you feel is best. If they have died, you can still forgive. Forgiveness is always for you, not the other person. Remember to forgive yourself. That can be the toughest part. Forgive yourself anyway.

Step Thirty-three

Soy: A Marketing Dream Come True

When I was in 6th grade, I remember reading about a farming process where plants were grown in a field for the sole purpose of plowing them under. That plant was soybeans. It was a natural fertilizer, adding needed nitrogen back into the soil. I remember thinking it was odd to grow something you weren't going to eat.

Times have changed.

When the food industry switched to polyunsaturated oils in processed foods, they discovered that soybeans gave a high yield of oil. And soybeans were really cheap! But there was a downside. The industry ended up with a lot of by-product called, soy protein isolate (SPI). So it was promoted as a health food and Americans bought it. (So did a lot of doctors and nutritionists.)

Here are some quick facts:

1. Soybeans are high in phytic acid, making it difficult for you to absorb calcium, magnesium, iron, and zinc. The phytic acid content can be reduced, but it takes a long fermentation process to do so.

2. Fermented soy products, like miso and tempeh, contain nutrients that are easily absorbed. Hemaglutinin, a substance that promotes blood clotting, is de-activated during fermentation.

3. Soy is very difficult to digest. It can cause bloating, gas, constipation, and diarrhea. It is not a good choice for those who already have colon or digestive problems.

4. Soy can adversely affect thyroid function. Most of us want our thyroid glands to be working up to speed since the thyroid keeps our metabolism at optimum levels.

5. Nearly all the soy on the market is Genetically Modified. That, by itself, is a good reason to avoid it.

Soy is not bad. But it is definitely not a medicine or a health food. Neither is it essential. Today, the way soy is refined and mass-produced, it is a processed food. And it is good for your health to avoid all processed foods.

Soy has definitely been miss-represented. And now it is a billion dollar industry. Soy is in *everything*. Keep reading those labels. Avoid soy.

Step Thirty-four

Meditation

Meditation is a way to quiet your mind. It takes deep breathing one step further by focusing on a word, and letting other thoughts waltz through your mind and move on their way while you focus on the word. It is relaxing and restful. Afterwards people feel rejuvenated. It is recommended that people meditate 15 to 20 minutes twice a day. But 5 to 10 minutes can be helpful. Pick a word, any word. I recommend the word "breathe." (You don't really need a word. Just focus on your breathing.)

Find a quiet place where you will not be interrupted. Sit in a chair, both feet flat on the floor. Close your eyes. Begin to breathe deeply. Think the word "breathe" as you inhale and exhale. As other thoughts come into your mind, allow them to move along. Don't push them out, just let them go. Come back to focus on your breathing and your word. Do this for 5 to 20 minutes, depending on how much time you have. This can be a great energy booster in the late afternoon, or once you are home from work. It can also help wake you up in the morning.

Do this on a regular basis for 30 days. You may find that you feel calmer, like you can just go with the flow. Little things don't upset you so much. Your fuse is not so short. Other people may notice you are more flexible; easier to live with, more relaxed. And then those minutes you thought were impossible to find to meditate, suddenly become a priority.

Watch Video: Patti Bowman, CN, talks about Step 34

https://www.authorpattibowman.com/step-34-meditation/

Step Thirty-five

There is More to This Than Gluten

The wheat we eat today is not the same wheat our grandparents ate. It has changed dramatically in the past fifty years under the influence of agricultural scientists. In the 50's and 60's, these scientists felt an urgent need to feed the world. They organized the International Maize and Wheat Improvement Center located east of Mexico City. In that climate, they had two growing seasons a year. This meant they could move twice as fast in their research. As a result of their efforts, we have 25,000 varieties of wheat today. For the most part, two varieties are now grown world-wide.

Modern wheat of today is the product of breeding to generate greater yield and characteristics such as resistance to disease, drought, and heat. Wheat has been hybridized to death—literally. Modern wheat does not grow in the wild. No animal or human safety testing was conducted on the new strains that were created. These products of agricultural research were released into the food supply without any safety concerns regarding human health.

Dr. William Davis, author of *Wheat Belly*, is very clear, that wheat has been altered by hybridization experiments. All this happened before genetic modification as we know it today. This is comforting, but not really. Because the author goes on to explain how wheat is adversely affecting our health. Wheat can spike blood sugar, can be addictive for some people, and stimulates appetite. It makes you want to eat more, especially wheat.

A couple of years after reading *Wheat Belly*, I read *Eat Wheat*, by Dr. John Douillard. Dr. Douillard claims that wheat is very healthy for us. It has a wonderful fiber that feeds gut microbes, helping us keep a strong immune system. That same fiber can shorten the time it takes for our meals to make their way through our digestive system and out of our bodies. These two books sound like they contradict each other. And they both contain scientific research to back up their claims. Now what?

Dr. Douillard goes one step further. He suggests we look deeper into the issue. He admits that wheat is difficult to digest. And in order for wheat to be helpful to our bodies, we must digest it and assimilate the nutrients. The question is how good is your digestion? In his book, *Eat Wheat*, he explains how to improve your digestion, improve the health of the microbes in your gut (known as the microbiome) and then maybe you can eat wheat again.

Both doctors agree that people with Celiac disease can never eat wheat. Some people with food sensitivities will feel better if they never eat wheat. Some people, when their digestive system has been strengthened, can eat wheat again.

Once your digestive system is strong, it is very important what kind of wheat you eat and how often. Douillard claims that fall and winter were the seasons that our ancestors would have gathered and stored wheat and other grains. He believes that is the time to eat wheat.

Besides a stronger digestive system, wheat also needs to be prepared properly. Wheat grains can be sprouted. They can also be soaked. When water and wheat flour are mixed together and allowed to sit, they lacto-ferment. Microbes in the wheat start to eat the sugars and the gluten. This lowers the content of both. Real sourdough bread needs a long (2 days) fermentation process. All you need is organic wheat flour, salt, water, and a starter. Our modern sourdough is processed within a few hours. Many additives are usually thrown in, including fats, sweeteners, and yeast. Read the ingredients to find out what you are really eating.

Ancient wheat, like einkorn and emmer, is much simpler genetically than modern hybridized wheat. Douillard says that is better for us. He also emphasized the need to use organically grown wheat. All the pesticides, herbicides and other chemicals sprayed on the soil or on our food, simply add to the total body burden, making it more difficult to have a strong digestive system and a healthy microbiome.

One way to figure out if this modern wheat is adversely affecting your health is to stop eating it for 30 days. I recommend that you replace the wheat calories with vegetables—rather than other non-wheat grains. Listen to your body! What changes do you notice? Would you like to strengthen your digestion? *Eat Wheat* has many suggestions for that. Consider placing both *Wheat Belly* and *Eat Wheat* on your reading list.

Step Thirty-six

Beauty is Skin Deep, Chemicals Go Deeper

Human skin is more than just a covering that keeps the internal paraphernalia intact. It is an organ. It is one way your body has to eliminate waste products. It helps regulate your temperature through perspiration. And it does offer a certain amount of protection. But it is not a raincoat. 60% to 80% of what you put on your skin is absorbed. Not exactly like eating, but close. When you eat, your liver gets first crack at the chemicals that come with your food, neutralizing them to protect your heart and brain. When you absorb chemicals through your skin, they go to the liver *after* affecting your heart and brain. So it is very important to learn to read labels.

There are thousands of chemicals in personal care products! Filtering through all the information can become overwhelming and down right depressing. Don't give up (or give in). A few basic ingredients to look for will give you a good clue as to whether to put it back on the shelf or not. This does affect your health in a big way, and also the health of your children.

Most of the chemicals come from petroleum—referred to as petrochemicals. One of these is *mineral oil.* When you do find it on the label, it is usually listed first. Mineral oil is also known as Vaseline, in other circles. Yes, I am afraid it is the same stuff. When you start reading labels you will be shocked at how many face and skin care products contain this ingredient. This is not something you want to put on your skin, especially your face! (By the way, baby oil is 100% mineral oil. NEVER put it on a baby!!) Mineral oil coats the skin somewhat like plastic wrap. Nothing can get in, but nothing can get out either—like toxins. This can slow down skin function, resulting in premature aging. And no one wants that!

Sodium Lauryl Sulfate (SLS) and *Sodium Laureth Sulfate (SLES)* are detergents. They can be found in 90% of personal care products that lather. Their purpose is to give you lots of suds, just like in the TV commercials. We have been conditioned to like lather. After all, if you don't have suds, you may not be getting clean! (Or so we think.) That is exactly what the industry wants you to believe. However, SLS (and its cousin, SLES) is a **known** skin irritant. It can easily penetrate the skin. It can also corrode hair follicles and slow down hair growth. Check your shampoo.

Propylene glycol acts as a wetting agent. This petrochemical has adverse health effects: skin inflammation, kidney damage, liver damage, skin rashes and dry skin. And that is just a start. It is also in anti-freeze, in case you want more of it than you can find in your body wash. Close cousins are *ethlylene glycol* and *butylene glycol.*

Parabens are next: *methylparaben, propylparaben,* and *butylparaben.* They are preservatives that also mimic estrogen in the body. This can disrupt the hormonal balance of your body. There is an association between breast cancer and prostate cancer and these estrogen mimicking petroleum by-products.

Polyethylene glycol (PEG) is a carcinogenic petroleum product that will reduce your skin's natural moisture, making your skin look older. Check your body lotion.

Diethanolamine (DEA), monoethanolamine (MEA) and *Triethanolamine (TEA)* are hormone-disrupting chemicals. They are restricted in Europe due to carcinogenic effects, yet are still used in the U.S. Americans may be exposed several times a day through shampoos, body washes and body lotions.

Triclosan is a synthetic chemical used in "antibacterial" products. The Environmental Protection Agency (EPA) registers triclosan as a pesticide, giving it high scores as a risk to the environment and people. It is found in antibacterial soaps and "water-free" hand cleaners. Triclosan and triclocarban interfere with your hormonal system. Triclosan interferes with the thyroid and triclocarban interferes with sex hormones, both female and male. These products are often available in schools for children to use instead of washing their hands with water. By the way, research shows that regular soap and water is just as good. Advertisers want us to be afraid of "germs" and buy their antibacterial products. And it seems to be working.

Even though triclosan has recently been banned in by the Food and Drug Administration, this ban is only for soaps, and manufacturers have a year to remove it. It can still be found in other products (like toothpaste), so keep reading those labels.

Sodium hydroxide is relatively new to personal care products. It may be fatal if swallowed. Check your toothpaste tube.

And then there are the 4,000 ingredients that come under the heading of "Fragrance." Not to mention the FD&C color pigments, mostly made from coal tar. "Fragrances" affect the nervous system. Colors can cause skin irritations. Some are carcinogenic.

To find all the above ingredients, look at labels on: baby wipes, diaper creams, baby lotion, facial cleansing cloths, facial cleaners, body washes, shampoos, toothpastes, shaving cream, body lotions, deodorants, hand lotions, antibacterial washes, soaps, etc. Even "natural" and "organic" products can contain these ingredients.

These products are used because they are cheap and few people are noticing. So if you don't want to apply chemicals to your face, teeth, and body several times a day, every day, look for something safer. There are many safer products available. Consumers always vote with their money. Make your vote count for health!

Step Thirty-seven

A Lump of Water

Did you know that you are about 70% water? With all your bones, muscles, and organs taking residence within, that is still a lot of water! No wonder that we need to drink a lot of it. Water doesn't just transport "stuff" through our veins; it has many other functions. Water cushions our joints, protects organs and tissues, carries oxygen to cells, regulates body temperature, helps produce digestive enzymes, and much more. I am not talking fluids, I am talking w-a-t-e-r.

According to Dr. F. Batmanghelidj, M.D., Americans have been led to believe that any fluid counts. He says this is a great misunderstanding. When the body wants water, it wants water. If you add anything to the water, it then becomes a food and gets digested. When you first get sick, think dehydration. Try water first before any medication. Dr. Batmanghelidj has spent many years studying the effects of water on health. You can read all about it in his book, *Your Body's Many Cries for Water*. In American culture, we have learned to reach for something else to satisfy our thirst: coffee, tea, milk, juice, alcohol, cola, sports drinks, etc. Yet these drinks can actually cause more dehydration. When water is what your body wants, water is what it wants. Remember, you are 70% water. (And your brain is about 80%!)

A lot of people tell me that they don't like the taste of water. Chlorine does not taste good. I agree. To get rid of that taste, you can boil the water. You can also set water out overnight and the chlorine will escape into the air. Then there is the option of a charcoal filter that takes the chlorine out. Also remember, if you have been drinking other fluids, instead of drinking water, your taste buds need time to adjust. Of course, water will not taste like a sugary drink. Drink water anyway. Give your body a chance to re-hydrate and some of your health issues may disappear. You don't see how there could possibly be a connection between your health issues and water? Read the book. It has sold over a million copies and has been translated into 15 languages.

Step Thirty-eight

Vitamin B-12

What do fatigue, dementia, dizziness, depression, mini-strokes, infertility, neuropathy, memory loss, heart attacks, blood clots, stomach pain, shortness of breath, and ringing in the ears all have in common? According to Sally Pacholok, R.N., B.S.N., and Jeffrey Stuart, D.O., all these symptoms (and more!) are related to B-12 deficiency. Their book, *Could it Be B-12?,* discusses all the issues surrounding B-12 deficiency and the problems with getting correctly diagnosed. The authors believe that the misdiagnosis of B-12 deficiency is epidemic. Many people suffer needlessly, especially those over age 60. Yet all ages can be affected.

Because B-12 affects so many body systems, a deficiency can look like other diseases. Doctors often attribute symptoms to pre-existing conditions like mental illness, aging, or MS. And as the authors point out, even when doctors do screen for B-12 deficiency, they usually use the serum B-12 test which is inaccurate. Pernicious anemia is the most well-known cause of B-12 deficiency, but not the most common. One third of people with a B-12 deficiency never develop anemia. Therefore their disease is not detected by routine blood tests. To be properly screened, you need to know the numbers on your test results. Do you fall in the "gray zone"? This is between 200 pg/ml and 450 pg/ml. Most doctors do not treat patients who fall in the "gray zone" even if they have symptoms. Knowing your score, you can request another test. This is the urinary MMA. These two tests help clarify whether you need treatment. You may have to insist. So be assertive! A third test is Homocysteine (Hcy). This test checks for B-12, B-6, and folate. This is important to your health and well-being. There is a window of opportunity to reverse your symptoms. If you wait too long, it may be too late.

The authors are trying to convince doctors that by changing the range on the serum B-12 test to a low of 450 pg/ml (instead of a low of 200 pg/ml), more people could be helped. But change is slow in coming. Knowing this information about B-12 could save your life or the life of someone you love.

Sources of vitamin B-12 in food include: eggs, dairy, meat, fish, poultry, and foods fortified with B-12. But just because you are eating foods with B-12 does not mean you are absorbing it. You don't need a lot of B-12 daily, but it does follow a complex pathway from your mouth to your cells. First, you need a lot of hydrochloric acid in your stomach to split the B-12 from the protein it is attached to. Your body uses other proteins to escort the B-12 into the small intestines, into the blood stream, and on to the cells. This complicated process can break down at any point.

Some people have an increased chance of developing this deficiency: vegetarians and vegans; people who have had gastric or intestinal surgery; people who often use antacids; those on diabetic drugs like Metformin; people who have had surgeries or dental procedures using nitrous oxide; people with a history of anorexia or bulimia; those with a history of alcoholism; those with a family history of pernicious anemia; people diagnosed with anemia of any kind; people with Crohn's, IBS, or celiac disease; people with autoimmune disorders; women with a history of infertility or multiple miscarriages; and infants born and breast fed by mothers who are deficient in B-12 for any reason.

More information is available in the book, including a more detailed symptom survey. This is really important! This health issue is easy to solve---cheaply!! It's up to you to find the answer. Read the book. Be informed.

Step Thirty-nine

Real Cows Give Real Milk

Real cows are the ones grazing on green grass. Their milk contains important nutrients, like vitamins A, D, E, K-2, C, B-6, and B-12. This is the milk where the cream rises to the top. That fat contains vitamins A and D, needed to assimilate the calcium and protein in the milk part. Nature intended real milk to give us great nourishment.

Along came pasteurization in the 1920's. Children were dying of TB, infant diarrhea, and other diseases. Pasteurization saved a lot of lives. But the problem wasn't really with the milk. The problem was the cows were undernourished, water supplies were infected, and production methods were filthy. Pasteurization was to be a temporary solution until those problems could be cleared up. It didn't work out that way.

Most people think pasteurization is necessary for safe milk. That's not true. Today, we have stainless steel tanks, milking machines, refrigeration, cleaner water, and much improved testing methods. Now it is pasteurized milk you want to avoid.

Pasteurization destroys enzymes, reduces or destroys nutrients, and kills the good bacteria. Calves fed pasteurized milk are not healthy and often die before they are fully grown.

Most commercial milk comes from Holstein cows. They are bred to produce a lot of milk and to survive on a grain-based diet instead of grass. Commercial cows are also fed soy meal, cottonseed meal, bakery waste, chicken manure, and other things you don't want to know about. Some are kept in confinement their entire lives and never see grass. And even though their pituitary gland is sending out high levels of growth hormone, they still may be given genetically engineered bovine growth hormone to push them to the limit of milk production. These commercial cows live 3 and ½ years on average before they become your hamburger. Real cows eating real grass live about 12 years.

For you women who have breastfed your babies, you know that what you eat ends up in your milk. It's the same for cows. And remember, it is this same milk that becomes your yogurt smoothie, pizza topping, ice cream dessert, and that blob of butter and sour cream on your baked potato.

Healthy real milk can be purchased from farms or through cow shares in many states. A few states have it available in stores. Check out realmilk.com for more information and sources near you. When you buy real milk, you support the local small dairy farmer and your health.

Step Forty

Fears-Don't Go There!

Mainstream medicine is based on fear. Fear of the unknown, fear of disease, fear of getting older, fear of "not catching it in time," fear of getting sick, fear of your family history, fear of your genetic code, and on and on and on. **Don't go there!**

Stop being afraid of every disease you hear about on TV. Remember, those companies are *advertising*. That means they are trying to sell you something you probably don't need. If you consider yourself healthy, and you are happy, and you are making healthy changes in your life, you are probably fine. Trust yourself to take good care of you. Trust your body to heal itself. It's very good at it, actually! When you do notice something unusual, then you need to go see your doctor. It is their job to figure out the problem. Whenever possible, focus on **health**. Focus on how good your body feels and how happy you are to be alive and enjoying life! Do not focus on fears of what "might" happen down the road. That kind of thinking will **not** keep you healthy.

Step Forty-one

Food Allergies

Food allergies are a complicated subject. There are food allergies and food sensitivities. To keep it simple, most food allergies give an immediate response. These are fairly easy to figure out. The response can be life threatening—anaphylactic shock. Headaches or breaking out in hives are other possibilities.

Food sensitivities (sometimes referred to as intolerances) have a delayed reaction. The response can take as long as 3 days to show itself. By then the person has had several meals, so deciphering the offending food is difficult. Many more people have food sensitivities than allergies. But most people don't realize they do. "So what?" you say. Because food sensitivities are an immune response to an "invader;" if you keep eating the offending food, you really wear out your immune system. Then you are more prone to illnesses. Food sensitivities keep many people from losing weight. Your liver is kept very busy trying to neutralize all these "invaders." It gets tired. Then its other jobs are compromised.

If you have any long-standing health issues, food sensitivities could be the culprit. Consider doing an elimination diet. You remove from your diet the most common foods that cause sensitivities, as well as any food that you eat a lot of, or crave. The top nine are: wheat, gluten, dairy, eggs, peanuts, tree nuts, soy, corn, and shellfish. Keep them out of your diet for at least 2 weeks. Thirty days is better. Then introduce them back into your diet, one at a time. (*Warning*: if you cheat during your 2-4 weeks, you have to start over!) You need to wait 4 days to see if you get a reaction before introducing the next food. Reactions can be anything: headache, migraines, runny nose, fatigue, upset stomach, feeling like you are going to be sick, joint pain, muscle aches, brain fog, lack of concentration, anxiety, irritability, skin outbreaks, etc. If you get a reaction, stop eating that food. If you don't get a reaction, remove the food from your diet until you have tested all of the "top nine." Then you can add back in the ones that didn't bother you. Keep the offending foods out of your diet for six months to a year. That allows time for your body to heal. Then introduce them again and see what happens.

Many people are inclined to say, "I just don't think I have food sensitivities," or "I really don't think it bothers me." The only way to tell is to remove the food from your diet and then reintroduce it later. Others will say, "I don't eat that much." But it is not about the amount. It is about the immune system's response. It only takes a tiny bit to activate the immune system! Just like it only takes a teeny tiny bacterium to activate your immune system. I am constantly amazed at the results of this experiment. Many people are taking medications for a condition that is related to a food sensitivity. They have no idea there is a connection. Others have "put up with" a condition for years that disappears once the offending food is found and removed from the diet. Some start to lose weight when nothing worked before. Give it a try. It's worth it!

Step Forty-two

Relax

We are always being told to relax. But it may be a chal-
lenge to find something that allows us to relax and process
the busy-ness of our lives. Meditation has already been covered in this book. That is something you can do every day
to release tension. Exercise is a great way to release tension, but you may not find it relaxing. Some people find a
warm bath very relaxing and soothing. Deep breathing can
also help you to "calm" those nerves. Five to ten minutes of
deep breathing every day can lower blood pressure. Massage Therapy can be a great way to relax. Not something you
would probably do every day, but it can help you let go of
the craziness. Just *thinking* about how great a massage will
feel, can help you get through a trying day.

Massage Therapy taps into your parasympathetic nervous
system—your restful state. Some people prefer a relaxation

massage. Some prefer something deeper to get tightness out of soft tissues. Either way, they usually feel more relaxed.

Some people find gardening relaxing. Others like to knit, carve wood, paint, sew, or some other craft they can do with their hands. Others will walk the dog and find relaxation just being outdoors.

Sometimes we relax by saying "no". Saying "no" can reduce the number of activities we have on our calendar. This allows us the time we need to actually chill out. Some people have a difficult time saying "no". They feel guilty, like they are letting others down. If saying "no" to someone's face is difficult for you, try this phrase, "I'll check my calendar and get back to you." This gives you time to gather your courage. It is a busy world out there. We have to pick and choose what is best for us, no matter how worthy the cause.

It is best to avoid TV as a way to relax. TV may numb you and render you "semi-conscious," but that does not really help you reach that parasympathetic nervous system.

Learning to relax is important for your health. It helps keep your world in balance. Think of something you find relaxing. Commit to making it a part of your day for 3 weeks. Then evaluate. Can you go with the flow more easily? Ask the people you live with what they think. You may need a combination of techniques to truly relax.

Step Forty-three

Fermented Foods

Years ago, before freezers or canning, people preserved foods using lacto-fermentation. Lactic acid is a natural preservative. It keeps the bacteria from spoiling the food. Many lactic acid-producing bacteria live on fruit, leaves, roots, and know how to take the starches from the fruits and vegetables and convert them to lactic acid. In the process, they provide a food with lots of enzymes, more vitamins, as well as probiotics, the friendly flora that keep our gut in good shape.

In Europe, sauerkraut was very popular. In Korea, kimchi is eaten on a daily basis. In Japan, pickled vegetables are served with each meal. Americans had corn relish. In India, people fermented fruit to make chutneys. Sailors at sea would often carry sauerkraut with them. Its high vitamin C content would keep them from getting scurvy.

Salt is used to discourage the bacteria from rotting the food until enough lactic acid can be produced to preserve the food. Whey can also be used, to cut down on the salt. It takes 2 to 4 days (some take weeks) for the vegetables to sit at room temperature, depending on how warm or cold your house is. Then the jars of food can be placed in the refrigerator until used. They continue to ferment in the refrigerator, but at a much slower pace.

Lacto-fermented vegetables and fruits are meant to be eaten as a condiment. A tablespoon or two with your meat will help you digest it better.

Lacto-fermented vegetables are easy to make. There are websites with recipes and more information. Check out westonaprice.org or bodyecologydiet.com to get started. You can also find them in the grocery store, but be careful. If they have been pasteurized, the benefits have been killed off with the heating process. It's better to make your own.

If fermented veggies don't excite you, think about this. Learning about the microbiome is an exploding science right now. No one really paid much attention to these microbes that live in our gut (the microbiome) until recently. We have more microbes in our gut than we have cells in our body. Really! A lot more. The healthiest people have the most diverse microbiome. These microbes heavily influence our immune system. They feel when we are stressed out. Keeping them fed and healthy is very important to our overall health. Fermented vegetables are very important to that process.

Lacto-fermented vegetables have a sour/salty taste. Some people call it "tangy." For Americans who are used to foods being very sweet, you may not like them at first. Buy some at the store, and start with 1 teaspoon eaten with your meal. Work your way up to a tablespoon. In no time at all, you may develop a taste for them. You may even want to try making them yourself. It's something your body will love you for!

Watch Video: Patti Bowman, CN, talks about Step 43

https://www.authorpattibowman.com/step-43-fermentation/

Step Forty-four

Politics

Most of us are adult enough to know that every organization has its politics. The field of scientific research is not exempt. To me science should be quite clear, so there is no doubt. That's why there is a protocol to follow when doing research. But it doesn't always turn out that way. People are not perfect, and they are the ones doing the research. Sometimes a theory forms a scientific foundation, but has not really been proven beyond any doubt. When it comes to health, the public is often confused by research findings. Some "behind the scenes" information may be helpful.

There is some really good research being done. Sometimes it gets published, sometimes not. There is some "junk" research being done. ("Junk" research is defined as poorly planned, or they simply did not follow scientific protocol.) Some of it gets published, some of it doesn't. Doctors, who want to keep up on the latest in their field, are always look-ing at research—usually published in peer-reviewed medical journals. However, they rarely read the entire article. They really don't have time. So they read the conclusions. And sometimes, the conclusions are not supported by the body of the work.

Peer-reviewed journals contain articles that should be read by a number of doctors before they are ever consid-ered for print. It's a great idea in theory. But most of the time, those articles that are chosen, are read by two editors, and that is all the review they get. If the editors have a bias, then your research may not get selected, even though it is innovative. Plus, pharmaceutical companies advertise in the medical journals. They let their voice be heard if a piece of research makes their product look bad. They put pressure on editors to have a certain bias or they will remove their advertising.

Pharmaceutical companies do most of their own research. Let's say they do ten studies. Five make their product look good, so they publish those five. But the other five make their product look bad, so they only publish one. Then a doctor, trying to give patients the best care, looks at all the research and decides this must be a good product, based on the six studies. The doctor may not even *know* that other studies were done. It is pretty hard to do your job well if you don't have all the facts.

And then there is "ghost writing". This has become very popular in the past 10 to 15 years. An example is a pharma-ceutical company that has a product they want to sell. They hire someone (usually in-house) to write the research paper.

Then they contact research doctors or scientists in the field, and pay them to put their name on the paper, thus giving the research credibility. These research papers are written so well that no editor (or doctor) can tell the difference. When they get published, no one knows that the person whose name is on the paper had nothing to do with the research. Editors are aware of this problem, but time constraints do not allow them to follow up in every case.

You could do some amazing research; but, if your topic is unpopular, you won't get any funding. Scientific research topics come and go like fashions. So if you happen to be working on something that is "in," lucky for you. But if it's "out" or worse, seen as ridiculous by your peers, you are out of a job. It doesn't matter how innovative you are.

Despite all these road blocks, careful, innovative research does manage to get through. So when you hear about this or that research, one good question to ask is "Who funded the research?" Mostly, just keep an open mind. Science isn't always so scientific. Sometimes it is just political.

Step Forty-five

Step Forty-five

People Need People

We Americans like to think of ourselves as independent. But when it comes to health, those who have a support network of friends and family are healthier, live longer, and live happier. Not your family? Okay, not every family is supportive. Not all friends are supportive. As an adult, you can choose to gather around you those people who love and accept you just the way you are. These are the people who will come to your aid in a crisis and be there to celebrate your successes. Whether it is through genes, work, a special club, a church, volunteering, or some other organization, we all have fuller lives when we have relationships with people who care about us and we care about them. We need each other.

If you don't have such a group, now is the time to start building one. It may take some time, so don't put this off. Start networking. Go where you feel most comfortable and start sharing yourself. Take time to get to know the people in your target group. Let them get to know you! It may be awkward at first, but the rewards will be worth it.

Step Forty-six

Beliefs

Everyone has beliefs. We pick them up along our journey through life. We have beliefs regarding money, spirituality, our own worth, the worth of others, education, what is most important, and, of course, health. When it comes to health, we hear messages like: no pain, no gain; after 40, you start to fall apart; women gain weight after the first child; women gain more weight after the second child; it runs in my family; my parents had that, I probably will too; my joints ache, I must be getting old; growing old is not any fun; and on and on and on. We say it all the time, we hear it all the time, and sometimes it becomes a self-fulfilling prophesy.

Then there are other beliefs that simmer just under the surface, in what we call our subconscious mind. These are the beliefs that cause us to offer a knee-jerk reaction. We don't know why, we just "feel" that way. Finding these hidden beliefs is like being on an archeological dig. We are not sure what we will find, but it will be familiar. Most people are not interested in unearthing anything in their subconscious. But these hidden beliefs can give us clues to our health, or lack thereof--- as well as clues to other areas of our life. As we sift through, we can make a conscious decision as to whether a particular belief is working for us now. And we can decide to keep it, throw it out, or replace it with something that works better for us. It is quite an adventure, with lots of surprises!

Paying attention to our thoughts helps us discover our beliefs. Just remember, you are connected to every cell in your body and they are all listening to you. Sending the message that you are "going downhill" is not a wise move. Instead, try using some of the techniques in this book: journaling, affirmations, and visualizing yourself in better health. "Every day I am doing something to promote better health," is more uplifting than "I am getting old." Awareness comes first. Once you are aware, delete the old message or belief, and replace it with a new one.

Step Forty-seven

Think Outside the Box

When people have health issues (mental or physical), they usually first go to a medical doctor. This makes sense. Medical doctors know a lot about the body. They know how to look for disease and how to treat it with drugs and surgery. That is their expertise. But if you are not getting answers, or don't like the answers you are getting, don't give up. Try going outside the box. There are many perspectives regarding health and what it should look like. Chiropractors are experts on the spine. If you are having trouble with your neck or back, they can do a great job for you. Some people just need someone to talk to and a mental health therapist can teach them valuable coping skills. These skills will be used throughout life. Some people manipulate energy. Rieki is one such practice. This is a very different perspective than allopathic medicine. Then there is hypnosis, which can help some people stop smoking. Others get help with weight loss.

Acupuncture is more "eastern" medicine. Needles are used to open up pathways in the body so healing can take place without interference. Nutritionists and Naturopathic Doctors help the body make positive shifts using nutrient supplements, nourishing foods, and lifestyle changes. Not everyone benefits from these "outside the box" perspectives. (Not everyone benefits from mainstream medicine, either.) But it is helpful to try different things. You may be surprised!

You may want to do some research first. Don't just depend on the Internet. Talk to friends and others who have experienced benefits (or not) from these modalities. Ask what they liked about it and what they didn't like. Ask for referrals. Don't be afraid to shop around. Sometimes when we step outside the box, a whole new world can open up for us!

Brent E. Smith D.C.—Step 47

**Watch Video Message from
Brent E. Smith, D.C.**

https://www.authorpattibowman.com/step-47-brent-e-smith-d-c/

Brent E. Smith, DC, has been in practice since graduation with a Doctorate in Chiropractic from the University of Western States in 2001. He specializes in Applied Kinesiology. He is a member of both the State and National Chiropractic Organizations as well as the International College of Applied Kinesiology. He is licensed in the State of Oregon.

Dr Smith lives in South Salem with his wife of twenty years and their two children. In his free time, he relishes spending time with his family. Their family activities include vegetable gardening, camping and fishing. He also likes to run and has successfully completed two marathons. Dr Smith also enjoys working with the Boys Scouts of America organization, helping young men attain their goal of becoming Eagle scouts. In his youth, he earned a second degree black belt in martial arts.

Currently, Dr Smith enjoys honing his public speaking skills with Toastmasters, and practicing his Spanish speaking skills.

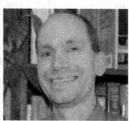

You can reach Dr. Smith at 503-378-0068 and learn more at his website: http://www.cppcsalemor.com

Brent E. Smith, D.C.

Dr. Manuela Terlinden—Step 47

Watch the Video Message from
Dr. Manuela Terlinden

https://www.authorpattibowman.com/step-47-dr-manuela-terlinden/

Manuela received her license as a naturopath in Germany in 1995 and specialized in acupuncture and Chinese Medicine. She ran her clinic for five years before a unique job offer in Hawaii prompted her to come to the States in 2001. At the same time, she got married and later settled down with her new family in Salem in 2006. After a diagnosis of cancer, Manuela had to reevaluate the focus of her life and decided to go back to school since her naturopathic license was not recognized here. In 2013 she graduated with a Masters in acupuncture and a doctor in Chinese medicine at OCOM in Portland, Oregon. She is a licensed acupuncturist in the State of Oregon and a board-certified herbalist.

Manuela says:"It has always been important to me that patients feel empowered by the healthcare they are receiving. The practitioner is the advocate for the patient, facilitating the journey to heal in a more holistic and complete way. Acupuncture nudges the self-healing power and generates balance. Healing is not just about symptom removal but to find the root of the disorder. It is a path where we re-discover what we need to live a balanced life. Patients are invited to participate in their healing process. In the end it is you who makes the change!

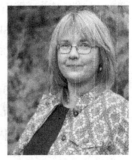

Dr. Terlinden can be reached by phone: 503-881-8996; through email: lifebalanceacupuncture@gmail.com; or at her website: www.acupuncturelifebalance.com.

Dr. Manuela Terlinden

Step Forty-eight

Honesty

To me, being honest is the first step toward healing your body of anything. Most people are honest with each other. They are not, however, honest with themselves. In other words, we lie to ourselves all the time. We say things like, "it doesn't matter" when it really does. We down-play our own needs so as not to inconvenience anyone. We talk ourselves out of things we want. We dismiss our feelings so often that we don't recognize a feeling when it shows up. We really want to say "no" but say "okay" instead, just to keep the peace.

In order to heal, we have to be honest about how we feel at every level. Do we really want to heal or is there a payoff for getting sick? Some people get sick so they can rest. Their body wants them to slow down, but for whatever reason, they are unable to listen to their body or "take a hint." Being sick allows them to go to bed and get the rest that they need.

Some people are resistant to answers to their health questions. They don't like the answer, so they refuse to believe there is a problem. It is easier to blame something else—like our age or our genes. Being honest with ourselves is not easy. It can take some sleuthing in the subconscious mind. But it is an important component in the journey toward wholeness.

How honest are you with yourself? Ask a trusted friend what they think.

Step Forty-nine

Information vs. Advertising

Most of the health information in the U.S. comes from television *advertising*. And because we hear it over and over again, we start to believe it is fact. I remember learning about the power of advertising back in High School. The best "commercial" has some emotional content that leads you to the conclusion that you need a particular product. I remember being surprised to discover that the advertisers did not have to be honest, either. (At least not until they get caught.) Then there were the "jingles," those little phrases, repeated over and over again, with or without music. You know, the ones that stick in your head, even years later.

Everyone in business deserves to advertise. That is why it is important for consumers to be aware. Advertisers are trying to sell you something. Before buying, learn about the product and the company. You want to be happy with your purchase.

Then there is the behind the scenes advertising that most consumers are not aware of. This is where the media comes in. We like to think that what is on the news is the straight scoop, that the reporters have researched their topics. But often, what you hear is a press release. (Press releases are written by the advertisers.) But you are not told that. Information you do hear is often bent to make advertisers look good. Who is advertising on this program? Those people are paying a lot of money to be heard. And they will not take kindly to a news release that makes them look bad. They will take their advertising dollars elsewhere. TV stations know that.

Rule of thumb: When you hear nutritional advice from TV, take it with a "grain of salt." It most certainly will be confusing, and probably not totally true.

Step Fifty

Tapping-EFT

I learned about tapping (also called Emotional Freedom Technique) many years ago, and recently have been re-acquainted with the concept. Ancient Chinese medicine is based upon energy or "chi" and how it flows through the body along meridians. This is the basis for acupuncture, placing needles along these meridians to get the "chi" flowing and thus bring the body into balance. Tapping utilizes these same meridians, but no needles. People simply tap with their fingertips on acupressure points to help themselves release physical pain, anxiety, fear, guilt, anger, sadness, or whatever is bothering them at the moment. It is a simple technique. Anyone can learn it, including children. And it is free.

If you are seeing a counselor or therapist, you could add tapping to what else you are doing. Or you can just try it on your own. What I like about the technique is that it empowers people to work out their own issues, instead of feeling helpless or like a victim. We have a lot more power than we think! This is one way we can help our bodies do what they are designed to do—heal.

I know this sounds a little crazy. There really is a science behind this. Just give it a try. You have nothing to lose and so much to gain. And it's free. (I think I said that.) If you have food cravings, try tapping about it. If you feel addicted to something, try tapping about it. If you hate exercise, try tapping about it. Really. Anything is game. Give it a go!

Brad Yates—Step 50

....

Watch Video Message from Brad Yates

https://www.authorpattibowman.com/step-50-brad-yates/

Brad Yates is known internationally for his creative and often humorous use of Emotional Freedom Techniques (EFT). Brad is the author of the best-selling children's book, *The Wizard's Wish*, the co-author of the best-seller, *Freedom at Your Fingertips*, and a featured expert in the film, *The Tapping Solution*. He has also been a presenter at a number of events, including Jack Canfield's *Breakthrough to Success*, has done teleseminars with "The Secret" stars Bob Doyle and Dr. Joe Vitale, and has been heard internationally on a number of internet radio talk shows. Brad also has over 700 videos on YouTube, that have been viewed over 17 million times, and is a contributing expert on the Huffington Post. More info is available at www.tapwithbrad.com.

The Wizard's Wish can be found: http://www.bradyates. net/ww/wizardswish.html
Freedom at Your Fingertips can be found: http://fayf.com/
The Tapping Solution film: https:// www.thetappingsolution.com/
BONUS VIDEO at YouTube: "Tapping for Kids-EFT with Brad Yates (and friends)"   http://bit. ly/2xwS3HM

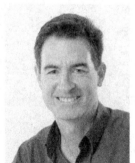

Brad Yates

Step Fifty-one

Giving Back

People who help others are healthier. Why? They feel good when they help out. Whether it is helping your neighbor, Habitat for Humanity, the local food bank, a lost child, giving up your seat on the subway, or cleaning up a mile of freeway, contributing to the community where we live, feels good. Yes, we often give our money, but when we give a piece of ourselves, our time, and our expertise, that is when we reap the benefits of joy that convert into wholeness. Happy people are healthier.

Where would you like to help out? Opportunities are endless and enterprising folks are creating new ones all the time. Volunteer! You can bring a "smile" to your life as well as someone else's. You get paid in appreciation. That's a real health booster!

Step Fifty-two

Choices, Choices, Choices

One of the great things about being human is the ability to choose. We can choose how we feel. We can choose what to think about. We can even choose what we want. In a world where we may wonder if we have any control at all, there are plenty of choices to be made. Sometimes the possibilities are overwhelming.

How healthy we are is a choice we make. We decide what we put in our mouths. We decide how much sleep to get. We decide to skip exercising today. We decide to quit smoking. We choose to make changes, or just keep doing the same old things we have always done. Some people are motivated by pain, some by illness, and some by a heart attack. With some folks, nothing motivates them at all! Part of the problem is that often the information we get is confusing, contradictory or unreliable. We don't know to whom we should listen, so we stop listening all together. That's still a choice.

We can be pro-active or re-active---our choice. How do you want to feel 10--20--30 years from now? Choose to invest in healthy living now and reap the rewards of your efforts later. (It's kind of like monetary investments.) Choose health now, so that later you have more choices.

Finale

Off and Running

First of all, make a list of all your bodily complaints. What bugs you about your health? What changes do you wish were possible? Write down every little tiny thing! Now go through the following check-list and mark off all the things you already do. Congratulate yourself for getting this far! Find one or two you would like to start on next. Come up with a plan. Decide on a date to start. Decide on a date to finish. Find a friend or group of friends to do this with. Be accountable to each other. Encourage each other. Some changes will require opening up your mind to new ideas or possibilities. Others will require more courage or grit. Celebrate each step! You are taking charge of your own health, your own life. Congratulations! You are on your way!!

Watch Video: Patti Bowman, CN, concludes the book

....

https://www.authorpattibowman.com/52-ways-finale/

Check-list

1. Make a list of all your bodily complaints. Keep the list in a safe place.

2. Stop smoking

3. Stop drinking soda pop

4. Exercise

5. Make a list of things you love to do. Do one (at least!) every week.

6. Sit down when you eat. Chew. Focus on the food.

7. Become a label reader

8. Delete High Fructose Corn Syrup from your diet

9. Make a list of things you appreciate about yourself. Practice accepting compliments. Appreciate yourself and others more.

10. Avoid MSG

11. Delete artificial sweeteners from your life.

12. Start a Journal. Keep it up for 3 weeks.

13. Switch to unrefined salt

14. Listen to your thoughts. Practice saying kind things to yourself.

15. Get in bed by 10 pm, every day for a week.

16. Visualize something you want to happen every day for two weeks.

17. Visit a local farm or farmer's market.

18. Remove GMO products from your diet.

19. Find something to laugh about every day.

20. Make a list of your life's successes. Congratulate yourself every day.

21. Eat healthy, organic fats at every meal.

22. Delete trans fats from your diet.

23. Start a gratitude journal. Keep it up for at least 3 months.

24. Take a sunshine break every day. Even five minutes.

25. Post an affirmation on the bathroom mirror. Say it out loud morning and night for 3 weeks.

26. Reduce caffeine intake. Consider quitting.

27. List your dreams. Pick one. Take one tiny step in that direction.

28. Switch to organic foods. Start with fats. Add others when you can.

29. De-clutter your house. Start with a drawer, cupboard or shelf. Don't forget the garage and attic. Hire someone to help if you need to. Do enough to feel the difference.

30. Reconsider your alcohol intake. Find an organic wine.

31. Try five new-to-you healthy foods.

32. Try some grass-fed beef, lamb, or bison. Try it more than once.

33. Forgive someone. Forgive yourself.

34. Remove soy from your diet.

35. Learn to meditate. Do it 1 or 2 times a day for a full month.

36. Eat gluten free for 30 days. Keep track of the changes you feel.

37. Read all the labels on your skin care products. Research more natural replacements. Replace all the kids' products. Replace as many of your own as you can.

38. Drink water whenever possible.

39. If you or someone you love has any symptoms of B-12 deficiency, see that testing is done.

40. If you choose to drink milk, make sure it is free of hormones. Consider researching cow share programs near you. Try goat milk as an option.

41. Focus on good health.

42. Consider food sensitivity testing or an elimination diet.

43. Find something relaxing and do it every day.

44. Try some fermented vegetables. Give yourself a chance to adapt.

45. Be aware of the bias and politics that influence scientific research.

46. Start building a network of friends.

47. Make a list of your beliefs about life, money, health. How are they working for you? Would you like to replace any?

48. Try an alternative medicine practitioner.

49. Be honest with yourself about one thing.

50. Analyze something you hear on the news. Do some research. Is there another opinion that wasn't given?

51. Go to youtube.com and learn to tap. Tap once a day for 3 weeks.

52. Volunteer somewhere for a day, or half a day. How did it feel?

53. For one week, keep track of all the healthy choices you make.

54. When you have completed this check-list, look at your list of bodily complaints. How do you feel now? What has improved? What is the same?

55. Take all the positive changes you have made, and continue them. Now you have a new lifestyle!

Resources: Good Reading for Better Health

These books, websites, and articles influenced my writing. You may find them helpful.

Adrenal Fatigue, James L. Wilson, N.D., D.C., Ph.D.

Breaking the Vicious Cycle, Elaine Gottschall B.A., M.Sc.

Clean Gut, Alejandro Junger

Clear Your Clutter with Feng Shui, Karen Kingston

Coconut Cures, Bruce Fife, N.D.

Complete Candida Yeast Guidebook, revised 2nd edition, Jeanne Marie Martin with Zoltan P. Rona, M.D.

Could It Be B-12? Sally M. Pacholok, R. N., B.S.N. and Jeffrey J. Stuart, D.O.

Drop-Dead Gorgeous, Kim Erickson

Eat Wheat, Dr. John Douillard

Excitotoxins, The Taste that Kills, Russell L. Blaylock, M.D.

Feelings Buried Alive Never Die, Karol K. Truman

Fifty and Fabulous, Zia Wesley-Hosford

Grain Brain, David Perlmutter, MD

Grain of Truth, Stephen H. Yafa

Heal Your Body A-Z, Louise L. Hay

Health and Light, John N. Ott

Hidden Food Allergies, James Braly, M.D., and Patrick Holford

Molecules of Emotion, Candace B. Pert, Ph.D.

Nourishing Traditions, Sally Fallon and Mary G. Enig, Ph.D.

"Nutrition News and Views" by Judith DeCava, C.C.n>, L.N.D. "Alcohol and Health" May/June 2002

Primal Body, Primal Mind, Nora T. Gedgaudas, CNS, CNT

The Autoimmune Fix, Tom O'Bryan, D.C.

The Biology of Belief, Bruce Lipton, MD

The Body Ecology Diet, Donna Gates, with Linda Schatz

The Coconut Oil Miracle, Bruce Fife, C.N., N.D.

The Tapping Solution for Weight Loss and Body Confidence, Jessica Ortner

The Yeast Syndrome, John Parks Trowbridge, M.D., and Morton Walker, D.P.M.

The Whole Soy Story, Kaayla T. Daniel, PhD, CCN

Salt Your Way to Health, David Brownstein, MD

Stress Effect, by Richard Weinstein, D.C.

Wheat Belly, William Davis, MD

Why Your Child is Hyper-active, Ben F. Feingold, M.D.

Your Body's Many Cries For Water, F. Batmanghelidj, M.D.

NongmoShoppingGuide.com

RealMilk.com

WestonAPrice.org

BodyEcologyDiet.com

TheTappingSolution.com

AmericanLungAssociation.org

About the Author

Patti Bowman has a variety of interests. As a Certified Nutritionist, she has great enthusiasm for healthy eating and healthy living. She understands that health is about the whole person. That means having fun, learning, and being creative also keeps you healthy. Her book, *52 Ways to Transform Your Health One Step at a Time,* reflects that understanding.

Patti now lives in Salem, Oregon. When she is not cooking healthy food, writing creative books for children, or creating journals, she has fun playing with art supplies. Watercolor and colored pencil are her current favorites. You can learn more about Patti's work here: www.authorpatti-bowman.com

Thank you!

Thank you for purchasing this book! I hope you have enjoyed it. You are now on the path to transforming your health. Please share your enthusiasm on FaceBook and Twitter.

I would also appreciate it if you would leave a short review of the book on Amazon. It will help other people know if this book is for them. Reviews also help me improve this and future books. If you have never left a review on Amazon, follow these simple steps:

Go to www.amazon.com

1. Sign in to your account. If you don't have an account, you need to create one to leave a review.

2. In the search bar at the top of the screen, type in "Patti Bowman". All my books should come up.

3. Click on the book you wish to review.

4. Under the title, you will see my name, the stars, and the word "reviews". Click on the word "reviews".

5. To the right of the bar graph, click on the words "Write a customer review"

6. Click on the number of stars you want to give the book, and write your comments.

7. Thank you!

Much gratitude,
Patti

Tweet about this book
Post to FaceBook

Other Books by the Author

Look for these creative books for children:

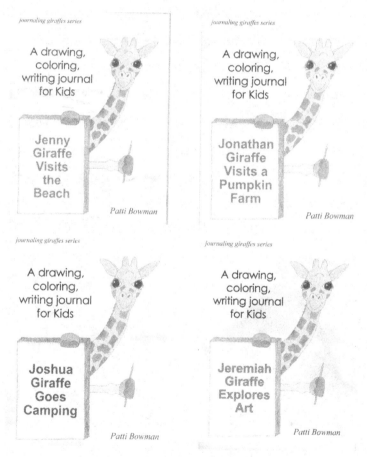

journaling giraffes series

A drawing,
coloring,
writing journal
for Kids

Jenny
Giraffe
Visits
the
Beach

Patti Bowman

journaling giraffes series

A drawing,
coloring,
writing journal
for Kids

Jonathan
Giraffe
Visits a
Pumpkin
Farm

Patti Bowman

journaling giraffes series

A drawing,
coloring,
writing journal
for Kids

Joshua
Giraffe
Goes
Camping

Patti Bowman

journaling giraffes series

A drawing,
coloring,
writing journal
for Kids

Jeremiah
Giraffe
Explores
Art

Patti Bowman

https://www.journalinggiraffes.com

CPSIA information can be obtained
at www.ICGtesting.com
Printed in the USA
FSOW03n0834111117
40952FS